Everyman, I will go with thee,
and be thy guide

William Harvey

THE CIRCULATION
OF THE BLOOD
AND OTHER WRITINGS

Translation by
KENNETH J. FRANKLIN

Introduction by
DR ANDREW WEAR

EVERYMAN
J. M. DENT · LONDON
CHARLES E. TUTTLE
VERMONT

This translation first published in Everyman in 1963

Revised edition published in Everyman in 1990
Notes © J. M. Dent 1963
Introduction © J. M. Dent 1990

This edition first published in Everyman in 1993
Reprinted 1996

J. M. Dent
Orion Publishing Group
Orion House, 5 Upper St Martin's Lane,
London WC2H 9EA
and
Charles E. Tuttle Co. Inc.
28 South Main Street,
Rutland, Vermont 05701, USA

Printed in Great Britain by
The Guernsey Press Co. Ltd,
Guernsey, Channel Islands

British Library Cataloguing-in-Publication Data
is available upon request.

ISBN 0 460 87362 8

CONTENTS

NOTE ON THE
AUTHOR AND EDITORS

WILLIAM HARVEY was born in Folkestone, Kent on 1 April 1578, the eldest child of Thomas Harvey and Joan Halke. He was educated at Kings School, Canterbury and at fifteen went to Gonville and Caius College, Cambridge where he took his B.A. degree, after which he began to study medicine. In 1600, he went to Padua where he studied medicine and anatomy under Fabricius ab Aquapendente, who encouraged his interest in embryology. After qualifying as a Doctor, Harvey returned to England and was admitted to the College of Physicians in 1604, the same year in which he married Elizabeth Browne. In 1607 he was elected Fellow of the College and, two years later, took up the post of Physician at St Bartholomew's Hospital. His famous work on the circulation of the blood was published in 1628. From 1618 Harvey had been one of the royal physicians; in 1630 he became Physician to Charles I and remained in the King's service until 1646, when he retired from public life. He published his work on the generation of animals in 1651 and died six years later aged seventy-nine.

KENNETH FRANKLIN (1897–1966) was formerly Professor of Physiology at St Bartholomew's Hospital Medical College. His translation of Harvey's *The Circulation of the Blood* was published in Everyman in 1963.

DR ANDREW WEAR lectures at the Wellcome Institute for the History of Medicine and has written extensively on Renaissance anatomy.

CHRONOLOGY OF HARVEY'S LIFE

Year	Age	Life
1578		Born Folkestone, Kent, 1st April
1593	15	Gonville and Caius College, Cambridge
1597	19	Bachelor of Arts, continues at Cambridge, probably studying medicine
1600	21	Padua University, Italy
1602	24	MD Padua, returns to England
1603	25	Plague Year
1604	26	Candidate and Licentiate of the College of Physicians of London, permitted to practise medicine in London

CHRONOLOGY OF HIS TIMES

Year	Artistic Events	Historical Events
1578		Francis Drake on voyage round the world
1583		William of Orange rules over Netherlands on defeat of the Spanish
1584		Sir Walter Raleigh discovers 'Virginia'
1588		Armada defeated
1589		Galileo Galilei professor of Mathematics at Pisa
c.1590		Dutch spectacle makers Hans Lippershey and Zacharias Jansen invent microscope
1593		
1597	Andreas Libavius' *Alchemia* (one of the first chemistry text-books)	
1600	William Gilbert's *On the Magnet*	
1601		English Poor Law system established
1602	Shakespeare's *Hamlet*	
1603		Elizabeth I dies, succeeded by James VI of Scotland and I of England. Hereditary shogunate rules Japan until 1867
1604	Hieronymous Fabricius ab Aquapendente's *On the Formation of the Fetus*	

Year	Age	Life
1604	26	24th November marries Elizabeth Browne, daughter of Dr Launcelot Browne, physician to Elizabeth I and James I
1607	29	Elected Fellow of College of Physicians
1609	31	Appointed Physician to St Bartholomew's Hospital, London
1613	35	One of the four Censors of the College of Physicians who regulated medical practice in London and prosecuted unlicensed practitioners; the appointment lasted a year
1615	37	Appointed Lumleian Lecturer in anatomy at the College of Physicians
1618	40	Appointed one of the royal physicians to James I

Year	Artistic Events	Historical Events
1605	Francis Bacon's *The Advancement of Learning*	Gunpowder Plot
1605–15	Miguel de Cervantes' *Don Quixote*	
1606	Ben Jonson's *Volpone*	
1607		Jamestown, Virginia, established
1608		Hans Lippershey invents telescope
1609	Johann Kepler's *New Anatomy*	
1610	Galileo's *Sidereal Messenger* (describing the moons of Jupiter seen by the telescope)	
1611	Authorised 'King James' version of the Bible	
1614		John Napier invents logarithms
1618		'Defenestration of Prague', start of Thirty Years War
1619	Johann Kepler's *Harmony of the World*	
1620	Francis Bacon's *Novum Organum*	Pilgrim Fathers leave in *Mayflower* to found Plymouth Colony, New England
1621	Robert Burton's *The Anatomy of Melancholy*	

Year	Age	Life
1625	47	A Censor of the College of Physicians
1626	48	A Censor of the College of Physicians
1627	49	One of the Elect of the College of Physicians with power to elect the President of the College
1628	50	*Exercitatio Anatomica de Motu Cordis et Sanguinis in Animalibus* Treasurer of the College of Physicians
1629	51	A Censor of the College of Physicians
1630	52	Physician to Charles I
1636	58	Physician to the Continental Embassy of the Earl of Arundel, meets Caspar Hofmann in Nuremberg
1642	64	Parliamentary troops plunder his London lodgings; loses his papers and drafts of books
1642–6	64–8	Often with Charles I during the Civil War
1645	67	Appointed by Charles I Warden of Merton College, Oxford to replace a Parliamentarian
1646	68	Ousted as Warden of Merton College, Oxford when Parliamentary troops take Oxford

Year	Artistic Events	Historical Events
1625		James I dies, succeeded by Charles I
1627	Francis Bacon's *New Atlantis*	
1630		Building of Taj Mahal in India begun by Shah Jehan
1632	Galileo Galilei's *Dialogue on the Two Chief Systems of the World*	
1636		Plague Year
1637	René Descartes' *Discourse on Method*	
1638	Galileo Galilei's *Discourses on Two New Sciences*	Harvard College founded
1642		Beginning of English Civil War Abel Tasman discovers Tasmania and New Zealand
1643		Evangelista Torricelli invents barometer
1644		End of Ming dynasty and beginning of Manchu dynasty in China
1645		Oliver Cromwell defeats royalists at Naseby

Year	Age	Life
1647		
1648		
1649	71	*Exercitatio Anatomica de Circulatione Sanguinis* (comprising the two anatomical essays to Jean Riolan on the circulation of the blood)
1651	73	*Exercitationes De Generatione Animalium*
1652		
1653		
1654		
1655		
1657	79	Death on 3rd June 1657, buried in Hepstead in Essex

Year	Artistic Events	Historical Events
1647		Blaise Pascal experiments to show existence of vacuum Quakers founded by George Fox
1648		Peace of Westphalia ends Thirty Years War
1649		Charles I executed
1651	Thomas Hobbes' *Leviathan*	Otto von Guericke invents air-pump
1652		The Dane Thomas Bartholin demonstrates lymphatic system in humans (*De Lacteis Thoracicis*)
1653		Oliver Cromwell appointed Lord Protector in England
1654	Francis Glisson's *Anatomia Hepatis* gives a detailed anatomy of the liver	
1655		Christian Huygens designs first pendulum-clock
1657		First fountain-pen made in Paris. Leopoldo de Medici founds the Accademia del Cimento in Florence, the first formal scientific institution

INTRODUCTION

The discovery of the circulation of the blood was made by a deeply conservative man. Yet it has often been ranked amongst the early triumphs of the new science of the seventeenth century, the science created by Galileo, Descartes and Newton that overturned the authority of Aristotle and classical learning. In addition to guiding the reader through Harvey's treatise on the circulation of the blood, *The Movement of the Heart and Blood in Animals: An Anatomical Essay* (hereafter referred to by its standard Latin abbreviation, *De Motu Cordis*), this Introduction also attempts to resolve the paradox of conservatism and innovation which holds the key to our understanding of Harvey's work.

Harvey was an anatomist and an Aristotelian. Anatomy was an important growth subject in sixteenth-century universities, especially in Italy and crowds flocked to the public anatomies. The salaries and status of anatomy teachers increased through the century and universities vied for their services. Anatomists began to argue that their subject, and not philosophy, was the foundation of medicine. Padua, where Harvey studied, became the leading centre for anatomical research. The rise of Paduan anatomy began in 1543 when Andreas Vesalius published his massive work *De Humani Corporis Fabrica (On the Fabric of the Human Body)*. This systematically criticised the observational accuracy of the anatomy of Galen (c. 129–c. 200 AD), 'the Prince of Physicians after Hippocrates', whose extensive writings on all aspects of medicine had acquired authoritative status. Galen did not have human material available for dissection and therefore had to use apes and other animals. Vesalius pointed this out in his own book, which, he claimed, provided the first proper human anatomy. The anatomists who followed Vesalius at Padua continued to develop a more accurate structural anatomy based on the injunction of seeing for oneself, 'autopsia'. However, like

Vesalius they were far less adventurous when it came to the function of the parts of the body and repeated the opinions of the Ancients. In contrast to the creators of the new science of the seventeenth century, earlier anatomists adhered to classical theories and saw themselves as part of traditional learned medicine.

Towards the end of the sixteenth century there was a shift towards the methods and theories of Aristotle (384-322 BC) and away from those of Galen. Aristotle, the great authority on all aspects of philosophy, had also written at length on biological topics. Harvey's teacher in Padua, Fabricius ab Aquapendente, like Aristotle, had interests in embryology and comparative anatomy, and his emphasis on producing a general anatomical picture of specific organs using comparative anatomy was also Aristotelian. This approach was to be repeated by Harvey. Essentially, the shift towards Aristotelian methods represented a movement from one classical authority to another, whose writings had much in common. Later, when the leading figures of the scientific revolution constructed their new science, they explicitly rejected the philosophy of Aristotle, replacing his qualitative and vitalistic view of the world and life, shared also by Galen, with one that was mechanical and quantitative.

Before examining Harvey's *De Motu Cordis* in detail, it is useful to outline some of the previous ideas on the blood and the cardio-vascular system. Galen's view of the function of the blood gave no hint that the blood circulated. Galen had believed that venous blood was nourishment for the parts of the body and was attracted from the liver, the blood-making organ, as and when a part needed food. Additionally, the veins and arteries had different functions; the veins were full of nutritious blood whilst the arteries carried vital life-giving blood. The latter was composed of pneuma (air heated and refined in the left ventricle of the heart) and blood, and this was conveyed from the heart to the rest of the body by a pulsative power of the arteries. Given the functional differences between the venous and arterial systems, and the fact that only a small amount of the venous blood (most of it being used by the body) was carried from the right to the left ventricle of the heart, via 'invisible pores' in the interventricular septum, (the fleshy wall separating the ventricles of the heart), it was conceptually difficult to think of a general circulation of the same blood around the body. In the Renaissance when Galen's ƨtructural anatomy was being tested, Realdo Colombo, Vesalius's successor at Padua realized, amongst others, that the 'invisible pores' in the interventricular septum did *not* convey any blood across the heart. In his *De Re Anatomica* (1559) he also showed experimentally that blood moved from the right to the left side of the heart by means of a transit across the lungs. (The thirteenth-century Arabic writer, Ibn an Nafis and Michael Servetus, a religious writer and trained anatomist who was burned at the stake for heresy in Calvin's Geneva in 1553, had arrived at similar views about the pulmonary transit of the blood, but their ideas had no influence on other anatomists.) By the use of vivisections, Colombo was also able to elucidate the action of the heart. In contrast to Galen, who had stated that the active phase of the heart was in diastole when it sucked in blood, Colombo described the heart as acting in systole when it rose, contracted and forcibly expelled blood outwards. Colombo, nevertheless, did not envisage a systemic circulation of the blood and by the end of the sixteenth century most anatomists supported his views on the pulmonary transit of the blood.

Harvey announced his discovery of the circulation of the blood in 1628 when he published his *Exercitatio Anatomica de Motu Cordis et Sanguinis in Animalibus (The Movement of the Heart and Blood in Animals: An Anatomical Essay)*. But Harvey had worked on the cardiovascular system before 1628. In 1615, he had been appointed Lumleian lecturer by the College of Physicians with the duty of lecturing on anatomy and aspects of surgery. Fortunately, we possess Harvey's lecture notes for his 1616 course on the whole of anatomy and from them we can reconstruct a few of the steps leading to his discovery of the circulation. In these notes Harvey shows that he had confirmed Colombo's views on the pulmonary transit of the blood, and he also concludes that the heart acted as a muscle in systole with the ventricles contracting and forcibly ejecting blood outwards, rather than sucking it in during diastole as was traditionally thought. The circulation of the blood was briefly mentioned in a late addition to the manuscript of the lecture notes inserted, in Gweneth Whitteridge's view, around 1627. From Harvey's own recollection of events in *De Motu Cordis* it appears that he had the idea of the circulation of the blood around 1619.

De Motu Cordis itself is brief and to the point. Unlike other anatomical writers, Harvey was not concerned with citing other authors and disputing at length with them. Harvey's whole emphasis lay in demonstrating (in the sense of proving by sight and reason) two things: the action of the heart and the movement of the blood. The book divides naturally into two parts, and it has been suggested by Jerome Bylebyl that they were first written as separate treatises which were later put together to form *De Motu Cordis*, the first and earlier book on the action of the heart comprising the dedication to Charles I and chapters one to seven and seventeen, the second and later book on the motion of the blood being the Letter to Dr Argent and chapters eight to sixteen.

In the first half of *De Motu Cordis* Harvey discusses the contradictions that followed from Galen's views on the movement of air and blood to the heart. Galen viewed the function of the left ventricle of the heart as heating and refining the air coming from the pulmonary vein together with the blood that was transmitted through the 'pores' of the septum. Harvey points out that this meant that the products of this heating, 'sooty vapours', were allowed through the mitral valve to flow back along the pulmonary vein, whilst the same valve prevented blood doing the same. Harvey also wonders how the 'sooty vapours' going back up the pulmonary vein and air going down towards the heart were kept separate, and he stressed that if the pulmonary vein was opened neither air nor vapours were to be found, but only blood.

Harvey continues in a more positive vein, and describes in chapters two to five the action of the auricles and ventricles of the heart and the arteries. Since, as was well known, it was difficult to pick out the movements of the human heart, he vivisected frogs, small fishes and other cold-blooded organisms whose hearts moved more distinctly than those in warm-blooded animals. He also observed the hearts of dying dogs and pigs because their hearts moved more slowly. In chapter six Harvey makes it clear that he is drawing upon comparative anatomy in order to produce a general picture of how the heart worked in all animals. In chapters six and seven Harvey shows that the blood moved from the right to the left side of the heart through the lungs, and he acknowledges Colombo's work on the subject. Up to this point Harvey has not written anything radically new, though he was much more detailed and systematic than Colombo.

It is in chapter eight of *De Motu Cordis* that Harvey announces his discovery of the circulation of the blood. In a passage which has been hotly debated by historians, Harvey discusses how he came to think of the circulation. The Latin of the 1628 text is faulty and the emended text of the 1648 edition is little better, but the sense is clear enough. Franklin's translation has been altered in the present edition to convey the literal sense of the Latin (see p. 45) and to show how, in a very long sentence, Harvey ruminates about the factors that led him to the circulation. It was clearly the meditation on the amount of blood leaving the heart and the allied investigations which moved him to think of the circulation. Rather than being led logically by observation to conclude that there was a circulation, Harvey had a hunch that there could be one. Afterwards, as he writes, he found this to be true, and in chapters nine to fourteen he demonstrates that there was in reality a circulation.

Harvey made quantitative experiments which showed that far too much blood left the heart in a given time for it to have been used up by the body and replaced by the blood manufactured in the liver from the chyle produced from ingested food, as Galenic physicians believed. The quantitative argument suggested that blood must flow continually in a circle, otherwise the body would burst, but Harvey had to show the pathways involved. Since he was using a magnifying glass and not the newly-discovered microscope, he could not see the connections between the arteries and the veins. However, he showed that a connection must exist by means of a simple experiment with ligatures (see illustration on p. 16). Taking blood from the arm was a very common medical treatment and ligatures were often employed, so Harvey was turning a well-tried technique to his own purposes. He ligated an arm very tightly so that no arterial blood could flow below the ligature down the arm. He then loosened the ligature slightly so that arterial blood flowed down into the arm but the ligature remained tight enough to stop venous blood from moving up above the ligature. The veins in the arm below the ligature became swollen and this indicated that blood had moved down the arteries and then up the arm inside the veins, so there had to be connections which allowed the blood to travel from the arteries to the veins. The last part of Harvey's anatomical demonstration of the circulation was to show that the valves in the veins always directed blood back towards the heart and did not act, as Fabricius, one of the discoverers of the valves had believed, to prevent the extremities of the body from flooding with blood. (In old age Harvey had told Robert Boyle, the chemist, that thinking about the purpose of the valves in the veins had led him to the circulation of the blood[1]). After he had shown that there was a circulation Harvey is then able, in chapter sixteen, to point to previously baffling phenomena such as the rapid spread of contagion through the body and then explain them by the circulation. At the same time, the existence of such phenomena gave further support to the circulation. Similarly, in the last chapter (seventeen) Harvey adduces anatomical evidence, such as the greater thickness of the arteries close to the heart, which, he argues, have been constructed by nature to withstand the greater force of the blood near the heart. This, he feels, supports his findings on the action of the heart described earlier in *De Motu Cordis*.

The methods that Harvey used in *De Motu Cordis* involved the vivisection of a large number of different species, and comparative anatomy to establish a general picture of the action of the heart and the circulation which would apply to many animals rather than to one, man. In his use of comparative anatomy Harvey was influenced by Aristotle and Fabricius. More novel were the quantitative experiments he employed to measure the amount of blood leaving the heart, which have been taken to show that Harvey was the first modern biologist and exemplified the new experimental and mechanical approach to nature of seventeenth-century science. But this view fails to take account of the formative influence of classical thought on Harvey's discovery. Harvey believed in the ancient idea held by Aristotle and Galen that all parts of the body had been constructed with a purpose, and that nature did nothing in vain. This belief in final causes was anathema to the protagonists of the new science. He also adhered to a traditional, vitalistic view which held that life had special qualities over and above those of dead matter; he could never have agreed with Descartes' mechanistic analogy comparing the living body with a clock. The difference between the approaches of the two men can be clearly seen in their explanations of how the heart beat. For Harvey, the action of the heart occurred because of a pulsative faculty or power of the soul, whereas Descartes held the innovative view that the heart acted mechanically, rather like a combustion engine. Harvey produced a revolutionary finding, but he did not have a revolutionary philosophy.

The roots of Harvey's achievement are to be found in the

anatomical tradition of Renaissance Italy. He was concerned to give an anatomical demonstration of the existence of the circulation, in the same way that any other anatomical structure would be demonstrated. In the *Second Essay to Jean Riolan* (included in this edition amongst *Letters and Essays on the Circulation of the Blood*) Harvey made it clear that the circulation was something to be proved or demonstrated by the senses 'in anatomical fashion'. Although observation and experimentation were part of the new science, Aristotelian philosophy could also be observational (Aristotle was famous for his observation and dissection of animals) and could therefore be a proper philosophical framework for an anatomist. If Harvey owed his sense of observational precision to the traditions of Paduan anatomy, there can be no doubt that the influence of Aristotle on Harvey was a powerful one.

His Aristotelianism can also be seen in his emphasis on the primacy of the heart over all other organs (Galen had stressed the primacy of the brain). In chapters eight and fifteen Harvey bursts out in praise of the heart. It was 'the starting point of life and the sun of our microcosm', 'the site and source of warmth'. The blood, having given its life to the parts of the body, came back to the heart to regain its original perfection and did so 'by the natural, powerful, fiery heat, a sort of store of life, it is reliquefied and becomes impregnated with spirits and (if I may so style it) sweetness'. These images and the consideration of the heart's purpose were essentially Aristotelian and may well have led Harvey to concentrate on the heart. If the motivation to focus on the heart came from Aristotle, Harvey nevertheless makes it clear that his ideas on the purpose of the circulation were tentative and separate from his anatomical demonstration of the circulation.

Harvey's discovery of the circulation of the blood was not immediately accepted by everyone. James Primrose, a Galenist physician, wrote in 1631 a diatribe against it defending traditional ideas. When Harvey visited Nuremberg in May 1636, as physician to the embassy of the Earl of Arundel, he met Caspar Hofmann, an expert anatomist and professor of medicine at nearby Altdorf. Hofmann did not accept the circulation, and despite a public demonstration by Harvey, he remained unconvinced. Harvey's letter to Hofmann, which is translated in this volume, was written whilst still in Nuremberg in response to

Hofmann's disbelief. In it, Harvey emphasizes the visual nature of the proof of the circulation and how other clear-sighted onlookers had seen what Harvey himself had seen (the repetition of experiments to the sight of others was a seventeenth-century test for truth).

The major attack on Harvey's discovery came from Jean Riolan the Younger, a great anatomist in his own right, a leading member of the Paris Faculty of medicine, physician to Marie de Medici, and a fervent defender of traditional medicine. Riolan had probably met Harvey at court when he travelled with Marie de Medici on her visit to London in October 1638 to see her daughter, Queen Henrietta Maria. Later, when in Paris, Riolan published his *Encheiridium Anatomicum et Pathologicum* (1648) (*An Anatomical and Pathological Handbook*), in which he accepted part of the circulation but also tried to preserve Galen's teachings. Unlike Harvey, Riolan realized that the circulation of the blood had the potential to bring down the whole of traditional medicine, and his anxiety over this possibility clearly motivated his attempt to arrive at a compromise position. Riolan argued that in the aorta (the great artery leaving the left ventricle) and in the vena cava (the large vein leading up to the right side of the heart) blood circulated rather slowly, whilst in their offshoots, especially in the intestinal region, the blood did not circulate. Harvey replied in 1649 by publishing his two anatomical essays to Jean Riolan in the form of a small book: *Exercitatio Anatomica de Circulatione Sanguinis* (*An Anatomical Essay concerning the Circulation of the Blood*). These are included in the present volume amongst *Letters and Essays on the Circulation of the Blood*. In the first essay Harvey specifically shows that, observationally, Riolan's position was untenable for the blood in *all* the arteries had a force and an amount indicating the circulation. In the second, he ranges more generally, giving new experiments in support of the circulation, and emphasizing how his philosophy of knowledge was based on observation and reflected Aristotle's own position.

Perhaps the most interesting reaction to Harvey's work came from Descartes, whose own anatomical researches supported the circulation of the blood. Yet Descartes' mechanistic approach to the body led him to disagree with Harvey on the action of the heart. In the *Discourse on Method* (1637), Descartes argued that the heart acted in diastole, when its innate heat rarefied the drops of blood in its chambers and made them expand and eject particles of blood. In this instance Descartes' need for a mechanical beginning for the heart's motion made him set aside Harvey's detailed observational description of the heart's action which had shown that systole was its active phase.

By the 1660s the circulation of the blood was generally accepted, and for the English Harvey's discovery was patriotically displayed as an illustration of the acuteness of Englishmen. It was also seen as an emblem of the success of the new science. Harvey's book on the generation of animals published in 1651 was widely ignored, redolent as it was with Aristotelian doctrines. Harvey himself never agreed with the new philosophy. John Aubrey recalled him as saying of Francis Bacon, the philosopher revered by the founders of the Royal Society that '"he writes philosophy, like a Lord Chancellor" saide he to me, speaking in derision'. Aubrey added that 'he bid me goe to the fountain head and read Aristotle, Cicero, Avicen[na] and did call the neoteriques [those who believed in the new philosophies] shitt-breeches.'

In the end the paradox of Harvey and the circulation of the blood can be resolved. There was nothing in Harvey's conservative approach to preclude novel discoveries in anatomy. Ancient and Renaissance anatomists valued independent and critical observation and there was much in Aristotle's approach and philosophy to encourage Harvey to think of the heart and the circulation. The discovery of the circulation was a fact of observation for Harvey, and not the basis of a new philosophy. Like Harvey's successors, we also accept it as such and this allows us to integrate it into a contemporary scientific framework vastly different from that which guided Harvey.

---

[1] Robert Boyle wrote that he: 'asked our famous *Harvey*, in the only Discourse I had with him, (which was but a while before he dyed). What were the things that had induc'd him to think of a *Circulation of the Blood*? He answer'd me, that when he took notice that the Valves in the Veins of so many several parts of the Body, were so plac'd that they gave free passage to the Blood Towards the Heart, but oppos'd the passage of the Venal Blood the Contrary way: He was invited to imagine, that so Provident a Cause as Nature had not so Plac'd so many Valves without Design: and no Design seem'd more probable, than That, since the Blood could not well, because of the interposing Valves, be Sent by the Veins to the Limbs; it should be Sent through the Arteries, and Return through the Veins, whose Valves did not oppose its course that way'

Cited in Geoffrey Keynes kt, *The Life of William Harvey* (Oxford, 1978), p.28 from R. Boyle, *A Disquisition about the Final Causes of Natural Things* (London, 1688), p.157.

NOTE ON THE TEXT

Harvey's Latin was not polished and requires skill to translate into English. The first English translation of 1653 perhaps best conveys Harvey's sense, being closest in time to the original, but its English is now difficult to grasp. Professor Kenneth Franklin, who combined a career in physiology with an intense interest in seventeenth-century medicine (he also translated works by Fabricius ab Aquapendente and Richard Lower from Latin into English), produced a skilful translation which is clear to modern readers whilst still retaining Harvey's seventeenth-century nuances.

Movement of the
Heart and Blood
in Animals

Most Serene King!
    The animal's heart is the basis of its life, its chief member, the sun of its microcosm; on the heart all its activity depends, from the heart all its liveliness and strength arise. Equally is the king the basis of his kingdoms, the sun of his microcosm, the heart of the state; from him all power arises and all grace stems. In offering your Majesty – in the fashion of the time – this account of the heart's movement, I have been encouraged by the fact that almost all our concepts of humanity are modelled on our knowledge of man himself, and several of our concepts of royalty on our knowledge of the heart. An understanding of his heart is thus of service to the king as being a very special portrayal, if on a more modest level, of his own functioning. Placed, best of Kings, as you are at the summit of human affairs, you will at least be able to contemplate simultaneously both the central organ of man's body and the likeness of your own royal power. Accept, therefore, I most humbly pray your most serene Majesty, with your accustomed goodwill and graciousness, this new account of the heart. For to you, who are yourself the new splendour of this age, and indeed its whole heart, its central figure abounding in virtue and grace, we rightly refer whatever good obtains in this England of ours, whatever pleasure in our life within it.

Your most august Majesty's
most devoted servant
WILLIAM HARVEY

To that excellent and distinguished man
DOCTOR ARGENT
President of the London College of Physicians
and the Writer's particular Friend
as well as to the other learned Physicians,
his most kindly Colleagues,
the Writer's very warm greetings!

Excellent Doctors! On several earlier occasions in my anatomical lectures I revealed my new concept of the heart's movement and function and of the blood's passage round the body. Having now, however, for more than nine years confirmed it in your presence by numerous ocular demonstrations, and having freed it from the objections of learned and skilful anatomists, I have yielded to the repeated desire of all and the pressing request of some, and in this small book have published it for all to see. The booklet's appearance under your aegis, excellent Doctors, makes me more hopeful about the possibility of an unmarred and unscathed outcome for it. For from your number I can name very many reliable witnesses of almost all those observations which I use either to assemble the truth or to refute errors; you so instanced have seen my dissections and have been wont to be conspicuous in attendance upon, and in full agreement with, my ocular demonstrations of those things for the reasonable acceptance of which I here again most strongly press. Over many centuries a countless succession of distinguished and learned men had followed and illumined a particular line of thought, and this book of mine was the only one to oppose tradition and to assert that the blood travelled along a previously unrecognized circular pathway of its own. So I was very much afraid of a charge of overpresumptuousness should I have let that book, in other respects completed some years earlier, either be published at home or go overseas for printing unless I had first put my thesis before you and confirmed it by visual demonstration, replied to your doubts and objections, and received your distinguished President's vote in favour. If, however, I have successfully maintained my thesis with you and our College, distinguished as it is by learned men of such number and greatness, then I am quite sure that I have less to fear from others; nay, even that which came from you, because of your love of truth, to provide my sole comfort will come also, I hope, from all others possessing a similar philosophy. For true Philosophers, aflame with love of truth and wisdom, never find themselves so sage or so full of wisdom or so abounding in perception but that they cede place to truth from whomsoever or whensoever it comes. Nor are they so narrow-minded as to believe that our forebears have passed on to us any skill or knowledge so complete in all respects and perfect that nothing is left for the industry and diligence of others to accomplish. Very many, indeed, profess that the things we know are negligible in amount compared with those we know not. And Philosophers suffer not themselves to become enslaved and lose their freedom in bondage to the traditions and precepts of any, except their own eyes convince them. Nor, while swearing allegiance to Mistress Antiquity, do they openly abandon Friend Truth and desert her in sight of all. But, while regarding as credulous and empty those who accept and believe all at first glance, equally do they regard as dull and senseless those who do not see the things that are manifest to the sense, or acknowledge day-time by the light of noon. Hence their teaching is to reject equally, in their course of training, on the one hand the poet's tales and the rabble's absurdities and on the other the suspensions of judgment of the Sceptics. Again, studious, good and honest men as a whole never let their mind be so overwhelmed by feelings of indignation and envy as to prevent them from giving a fair hearing to proposals made on behalf of truth, or from understanding what is demonstrated to them. Nor do they think it degrading to alter their view if truth and a public demonstration so persuade them, or regard it as dishonest to desert errors, albeit most venerable ones. For they know very well that it lies within all men to err and to be deluded, and that many discoveries have been made through the chance learning of one person from another, of an old man from a young man, of a keen-witted one from a foolish one.

It was, however, dear Colleagues, no intention of mine, in listings and upturnings of names, works and views of anatomical authors and writers, to make display by this book of my memory, studies, much reading, and a large printed tome. In the first place, because I profess to learn and teach anatomy not from books but from dissections, not from the tenets of Philosophers but from the fabric of Nature. Secondly, because I consider it neither fair nor worth the effort to defraud a predecessor of the honour due to him, or to provoke a contemporary. Nor do I think it honourable to attack or fight those who excelled in Anatomy and were my own teachers. Further, I would not willingly charge with falsehood any searcher after truth, or besmirch any man with a stigma of error. But without ceasing I follow truth only, and devote all my effort and time to being able to contribute something pleasing to good men and appropriate to learned ones, and of service to literature.

Farewell, Excellent Doctors, and look with favour upon your Anatomist

WILLIAM HARVEY

INTRODUCTION

*In which is shown the relative weakness of previous accounts of
the movement and function of the heart and arteries*

It profits one who is pondering on the movement, pulsation,
performance, function, and services of the heart and arteries to
read what his predecessors have written, and to note the general
trend of opinion handed on by them. For by so doing he can
confirm their correct statements, and through anatomical dissection, manifold experiments, and persistent careful observation
emend their wrong ones.

Almost all anatomists, physicians, and naturalists hitherto
suppose, with Galen, that pulsation and respiration have the same
function, and differ only in that the former derives from the
psychic faculty, the latter from the vital one, while in all other
respects they are alike, both in the service they render and in the
nature of their movement. Hence these authors assert (as, for
instance, does Girolamo Fabrizzi d'Acquapendente in his very
recently published book on *Respiration*) that, since the pulsation
of the heart and arteries is inadequate for the fanning and cooling
of the blood, nature has fashioned the lungs around the heart.
Thus it is clear that whatever these earlier writers have noted
about systole and diastole, in connection with the movement of
the heart and arteries, has all been penned with an eye upon the
lungs.

As, however, the movement and constitution of the heart are
other than those of the lungs, and of the arteries than those of the
chest, it is probable that their respective functions and services are
equally otherwise, and that the pulsations and functions of the
heart and likewise of the arteries differ very greatly from those of
the chest and lungs. For, if pulsation and respiration serve the
same purposes, and if (as is commonly stated) in diastole the
arteries take air into their cavities and in systole expel sooty
vapours through the same pores of flesh and skin; further, if
between systole and diastole they contain air, and at any given
time air or spirits or sooty vapours, what answer can those

holding such views make to Galen, who wrote in his book that the arteries normally contain blood and nothing but blood, certainly no spirits or air, as one can readily ascertain from his experiments, and from his arguments in that book? And, if in diastole the arteries are filled by the intake of air (the greater the pulsation the greater the intake), then should you, with a large pulsation obtaining, immerse the whole body in a bath of water or of oil, the pulsation must at once be either much smaller or much slower, since passage of air into the arteries is made more difficult, if not impossible, through the surrounding mass of bath fluid. Likewise, as all arteries, deep as well as cutaneous, are distended simultaneously and at equal speed, how will air be able to pass so freely and rapidly through skin, flesh and body fabric into the depths as it will through the skin alone? And how can the arteries of embryos draw external air into their cavities through the maternal belly and the substance of the womb? Or how do seals, whales, dolphins and the whole cetacean tribe, and all the fishes in the depth of the sea, by the diastole and systole of their arteries take in and emit air in rapid succession across the immense mass of water? To say that they suck in the air embedded in the water and return into it their sooty vapours is not unlike a fiction. And, if in systole the arteries expel sooty vapours from their cavities through the pores of the flesh and skin, why not also spirits, which they say are contained in these vessels? For spirits are much more rarefied than sooty vapours. And, if the arteries receive and give out air in systole and diastole, as the lungs do in respiration, why do they not also do so when cut across in a wounding? When the trachea is so severed, the successive in and out movements of air are obvious. When, however, an artery is severed, one sees an immediate and continuous expulsion of blood, and no in and out movement of air. If the arterial pulsations cool and fan the parts of the body as the lungs do the heart itself, how is it commonly stated that the arteries distribute from the heart to the individual parts blood packed with the spirits of life, which foster the heat of the parts, rouse it when torpid, and so to speak restock it when it is low? And how, if you ligate the arteries, do the parts not only straightway become sluggish, cool, and turn somewhat pale, but also finally cease to be nourished? According to Galen, this is because they have been deprived of the heat which had previously flowed to all parts from the heart, since it is clear that the arteries transmit heat rather than cooling and ventilation from the heart to the parts. Moreover, how in diastole can there simultaneously be drawn spirits from the heart to warm the parts, and from outside means for their cooling? Further, though some assert that the lungs, arteries, and heart subserve the same functions, they also say that the heart is the laboratory of spirits and the arteries their containers and transmitters, but deny, in opposition to Colombo's view, that the lungs either make or retain spirits. In addition, with Galen, and in opposition to Erasistratus, they stress that blood, and not spirit, is the content of arteries. Such views are clearly mutually conflicting and contradictory, with the result that all are deservedly suspect. That the arteries contain blood and transport blood alone is obvious from Galen's experiment, and in arterial section, and in woundings. For Galen asserts in very many places that in the space of half an hour, from the opening up of a single artery, the whole of the blood will be drained off from every part of the body in a large, torrential outflow. Galen's experiment is as follows. 'If,' he says, 'you tie an artery in two places with a fine cord and cut the part lying between the two ligatures along its length, you will find nothing but blood inside.' And so he proves that it contains blood alone. From which we can argue in like manner as follows. If you find in the arteries (an experiment I have fairly often done in dead human beings and in other animals) the same blood as in the similarly ligated and opened-up veins, we can by the same argument similarly conclude that the arteries contain the same blood as do the veins, and nothing beyond that same blood. Some, while attempting to resolve the difficulty by stating that the blood is spirituous *and* arterial, tacitly concede that the office of the arteries is to distribute blood from the heart to the whole of the body, and that these vessels are full of blood. For spirituous blood is none the less blood. Indeed, no one denies that blood as blood, even that which flows in the veins, is imbued with spirits. Nay, if the blood that is in the arteries is turgid with a more copious amount of spirits, one must nevertheless regard these spirits as being equally inseparable from the blood as are those in the veins. And, as to the idea that the blood and spirits form one fluid (as do whey and butter in milk, or heat [and water] in hot water), with which the arteries are filled and over the distribution of which from the heart they preside, why, even this fluid is nothing other than blood. Moreover, if they say that the blood in the arteries is drawn from the heart through the diastole of these vessels, they appear to impute the filling of the expanding arteries to the blood in question and not, as earlier, to the surrounding air. For, if they say they are filled from this latter, how and when do they receive blood from the heart? If the suggestion is that it happens in [arterial] systole, the impossible will come to pass, namely, arteries filling while they are contracting, or filling and not increasing in volume. If on the other hand the suggestion is that it occurs in diastole, they will receive at one and the same time for two opposing purposes both blood and air, both warmth and cooling; which is improbable. Further, the diastole of the heart and of the arteries cannot be simultaneous, as they state; nor can the systole. For how can one of two so conjoined bodies, when they are simultaneously increasing in volume, draw from the other; or, when they are simultaneously contracting, receive from the other? In addition it is perhaps not possible for something to dilate (dilation being a passive process) while drawing another substance into itself unless it does so in the manner of a sponge, squeezed from outside, during its return to its natural shape. It is, however, difficult to imagine such a happening being possible in arteries. On the other hand, I think that I can readily and openly show, and have before this publicly shown, that arteries increase in volume because they fill up like bags or leather bottles, and are not filled up because they increase in volume like bellows. This, it is true, goes contrary to the experiment described by Galen in his book under the heading, 'That the arteries contain blood'. He exposes an artery, incises it along its length, and inserts a reed (or hollow pervious tube), thus ensuring that the blood cannot escape and closing the wound. 'So long', he says, 'as matters stay thus, the whole of the artery will pulsate. So soon, however, as you pass a ligature and knot it over the artery and the tube, thus clamping the arterial coats to the reed, you will cease to observe arterial pulsation beyond the knot.' I have not done Galen's experiment and I do not think it could well be performed in a living subject, because the blood would erupt too forcibly from the arteries; the reed, too, without a ligature will not close the wound, and I have no doubt the blood will leap out through the reed and beyond it. By this experiment, however, Galen seems to prove that the pulsatile power spreads from the heart through the arterial coats, and that the arteries during their dilation are filled by that pulsatile force because they dilate like bellows, and do not dilate because they are filled like leather bottles. The opposite to this is, in fact, apparent both in arterial section and in woundings. For the blood escapes from the arteries in forcible spurts and, even if the distance it travels is now greater and now lesser, the spurt is always in the diastole of the artery and never in its systole. From which it is clear that it is the force of the blood which causes dilation of the artery. For it cannot itself, while dilating, project the blood with such force, it ought rather to draw air into itself through the wound according to common statements about the function of arteries. And let not the thickness of the arterial coats mislead us into thinking that the pulsatile force comes from the heart through those very coats. For in some animals the arteries are no different from veins; and in the most peripheral parts of the human body, with the arteries finely subdivided (as in the brain, hand, etc.), no one will be able by looking at their coats to distinguish arteries from veins, for the coat of each is identical. Again, in an aneurysm resulting from wounding or erosion of an artery, the pulsation is exactly the same as in the remaining arteries, though the arterial coat is missing. The learned Riolan, in his Seventh Book, concurs with me in this. And let no one think that the function of the pulse and of respiration is the same merely because he sees the pulsations get more frequent, larger, and more rapid for the same reasons as does respiration, e.g. running, anger, bathing, or anything heating, as Galen states. For not only is the very finding (which Galen attempts to explain away) opposed to such a view, since immoderate feeding causes increase in size of pulsations with decrease in size of respirations, but in addition children exhibit frequent pulsations simultaneously with infrequent respiration. Similarly in fear, cares, anxiety of mind, and even in some fevers, the pulsations are rapid and frequent, but respirations slower. These difficulties and others of similar sort follow on accepted views of arterial pulsation and function; equally, perhaps, are statements about cardiac function and pulsation a complex of very many problems which it is not easy to disentangle. The heart is usually called the source and laboratory of the spirits of life, by means of which it dispenses life to the individual parts. They say, however, that the right ventricle does not make spirits, but is merely concerned with the nourishment of the lungs. Hence they explain the absence of a right ventricle of the heart from fishes (and, indeed, it is absent from all lungless animals) and assert that the right ventricle of the heart is there for the sake of the lungs.

1. How, I ask, when the structure of the two ventricles is almost identical, with the same make-up of fibres, 'armlets' of muscle, valves, vessels, and auricles, and in our dissection-subjects with similar dark, coagulated blood filling each; how, I say, when each behaves, moves, and pulsates in the same way, can we regard them as having been designed for such very different functions? If the three tricuspid valves at the entry into the right ventricle hinder return of blood into the vena cava, and if the three semilunar ones at the opening into the artery-like vein have been made to hinder return of blood; how, when a similar arrangement holds in the left ventricle, can we say that these valves have not been made similarly to hinder forward or backward movement of blood?

2. And as the valves are almost identically arranged in respect of size, form, and position in the left ventricle and in the right one, why do they say that they hinder egress and regress of spirits in the former, but of blood in the latter? The same sort of mechanism does not seem calculated to prevent equally effectively movements of blood and of spirits.

3. And as the respective paths and vessels correspond in size, that is, the artery-like vein and the vein-like artery, why may the one be regarded as having a private function, namely, nourishment of the lungs, and the other a public one?

4. And how is it likely (as Realdo Colombo noted) that so much blood is needed for the nourishment of the lungs? Since this vessel, that is, the artery-like vein, exceeds in size both femoral distribution branches of the descending vena cava, taken together.

5. And, I ask, as the lungs are so close, and so large a vessel is available, and the lungs themselves are in continual movement, what reason can there be for pulsation of the right ventricle? And what need for nature to add a second ventricle to the heart for the sake of nourishing the lungs?

When they say that the left ventricle draws material, namely air and blood, from the lungs and the right sinus of the heart for the formation of spirits, and likewise distributes spirituous blood into the aorta; that sooty vapours are sent back to the lungs through the vein-like artery and spirit forwards into the aorta; what is it that keeps the two streams separate? And how do the spirits and the sooty vapours pass in opposite directions without mixing or getting into disorder? If the mitral valves do not hinder exit of sooty vapours into the lungs, how will they hinder exit of air? And how will the semilunar [aortic] valves prevent backflow of spirits (in the subsequent diastole of the heart) from the aorta? And in general, how do they say that the spirituous blood is distributed from the left ventricle through the vein-like artery to the lungs without the mitral valves meanwhile hindering such movement? For they have stated that air enters the left ventricle from the lungs through the same vessel, but would have it that the mitral valves should hinder its return. Good God! How do the mitral valves hinder the return of air, and not of blood?

Further, as they have assigned a single, purely private function (that is, nourishment of the lungs) to the artery-like vein, which is a wide and big vessel, fashioned with an arterial coat, why do they strongly assert that the vein-like artery, with the coat of a vein, soft and lax, has been made for several functions (three or four, to wit)? For they will have it that the air passes through that vessel from the lungs into the left ventricle: they will similarly have sooty vapours pass back through it from the heart into the lungs: and they will have a portion of spirituous blood distributed through it from the heart to the lungs for their revivification.

If they will have sooty vapours and air (the former from the heart, the latter to it) transmitted through the same tube, I must reply that nature is not wont to fashion one vessel and one route for movements and functions so opposite, and that I have never seen such anywhere.

If they claim that sooty vapours and air respectively pass out and in by this route as they do through the bronchial tubes of the lungs, why, when we cut out or open up the vein-like artery, can we never find air or sooty vapours in our dissection subjects? And whence comes it that we always see that vein-like artery packed full of blood, and never of air, while we perceive air still present in the lungs?

If one performed Galen's experiment, and incised the trachea of a still living dog, forcibly filled its lungs with air by means of bellows, and ligated them strongly in the distended position, one would find, on rapidly opening up the chest, a great deal of air in the lungs right out to their outermost coat, but no trace of such in the vein-like artery or in the left ventricle of the heart. If in the living dog either the heart drew air from the lungs, or the lungs transmitted air to the heart, they should do so much more in this experiment. Indeed, were the lungs of the cadaver inflated in an anatomical demonstration, who would doubt that air would at once enter the vein-like artery and left ventricle were any passages available for it? So highly, however, do they rate this function of the vein-like artery, namely, the transfer of air from the lungs to the heart, that Girolamo Fabrizzi d'Acquapendente claims that the lungs were made for the sake of this vessel, and that this is their chief role.

But why, will you please tell me, is the vein-like artery venous in structure if it has been fashioned for the transport of air? Nature should rather use tubes, and ringed ones at that (like those of the bronchi), so that they always stay open and never collapse, and so that they remain completely empty of blood, and fluid causes no hindrance to the passage of air, as it obviously does when the lungs are in difficulties with their tubes packed or moderately filled with phlegm, giving rise to whistling and rustling sounds during our breathing.

Even less acceptable is the opinion which supposes that two sources of raw material (air and blood) are required for making the spirits of life, and claims that the blood oozes from the right to the left ventricle through invisible pores in the cardiac septum while the air is drawn from the lungs through a large vessel, the vein-like artery; that, accordingly, fairly large numbers of pores have been provided in the cardiac septum for the onward transmission of the blood. But, damme, there are no pores and it is not possible to show such.

For the substance of the cardiac septum is denser and more compact than any other part of the body except the bones and tendons. Assuming, however, the presence of openings, how (since both ventricles distend and dilate simultaneously) is it possible for one of them to suck something from the other, or – specifically – for the left ventricle to suck blood from the right one? And why should I not believe that the right ventricle calls spirits from the left one through the aforesaid openings rather than that the left ventricle calls blood from the right one? It is certainly strange and inconsistent that in the same instant blood is more fittingly drawn through obscure invisible channels and air through very widely open ones. And why, I ask, for the transit of the blood to the left ventricle do they have recourse to concealed invisible pores that are ill-defined and obscure, when there is so open a way through the vein-like artery? It is certainly a cause of wonder to me that they have preferred to make or invent a way through the solid, hard, dense, and extremely compact septum cordis rather than through the open vein-like artery, or even through the tenuous, lax, very soft, and spongy substance of the lungs. Moreover, had the blood been able to pass through the substance of the septum or to be imbibed from the ventricles, what need would there be for the small branches of the coronary vein and artery to be spread about for the nutrition of the septum itself? Most noteworthy of all is the following. If in foetal life (when everything is more tenuous and soft) nature has been forced to take blood across through the foramen ovale into the left ventricle [and] from the vena cava through the artery-like vein, how can it be likely that she transfers it so readily and easily in the adult through the cardiac septum, now denser with age?

André du Laurens (in his Book IX, Chapter XI, Question 12), relying on the authority of Galen (*De locis affectis*, Book VI, Chapter VII) and the experience of Holler, asserts and claims to prove that the watery fluids and pus of patients suffering from abscesses can be absorbed from the chest-cavity into the vein-like artery, pass to the left ventricle and arteries, and be expelled with the urine or the faeces of the bowels. Indeed, he recounts in confirmation the case of a person affected with melancholia who, after many fainting fits, was relieved of a paroxysm by the passing of turbid, foetid, and sharp-smelling urine. He finally succumbed to this sort of illness and, when his body was dissected, nothing comparable to the urine he used to pass was found in his bladder or anywhere in his kidneys. In the left ventricle and chest-cavity, however, it was present in abundance, and du Laurens claims that he had foretold such a cause of the affections mentioned. For my part, however, I cannot help but be surprised that, as he had divined and predicted that heterogeneous matter could be evacuated by the route in question, he could not or would not readily perceive or stress that blood could naturally be carried by the same routes from the lungs to the left ventricle.

From these and very many other arguments it is clear that the statements made hitherto by earlier writers about the movement and function of the heart and arteries appear incongruous or obscure or impossible when submitted to specially careful consideration. It will therefore be very useful to look a little more deeply into the matter; to contemplate the movements of the arteries and of the heart not only in man, but also in all other animals with hearts; moreover, by frequent experiments on animals and much use of one's own eyes, to discern and investigate the truth.

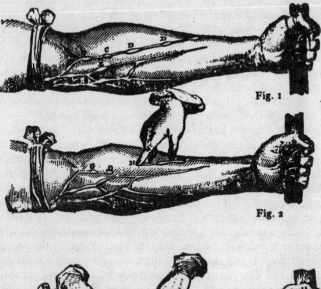

Fig. I

Fig. 2

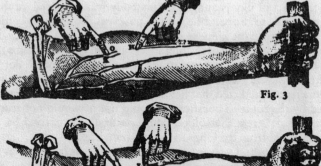

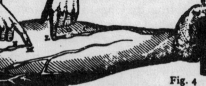

Fig. 3

Fig. 4

MOVEMENT OF THE HEART AND BLOOD IN ANIMALS
An Anatomical Essay

CHAPTER ONE
The Author's strong reasons for writing

When in many dissections, carried out as opportunity offered upon living animals, I first addressed my mind to seeing how I could discover the function and offices of the heart's movement in animals through the use of my own eyes instead of through books and the writings of others, I kept finding the matter so truly hard and beset with difficulties that I all but thought, with Fracastoro, that the heart's movement had been understood by God alone. For I could not rightly distinguish how systole or diastole came about, nor when or where constriction and dilatation occurred. This was because of the rapidity of the movement, which in many animals remained visible for but the wink of an eye or the length of a lightning flash, so that I thought I was seeing now systole from this side and diastole from that side; now the opposite; the movements now diverse, and now inextricably mixed. Hence my mind was all at sea and I could neither come to a decision myself nor assign definite credit to others. And I was not surprised that André du Laurens had described the heart's movement as being like Aristotle's concept of the flows and ebbs of the Euripus.

At length, through ever wider and more meticulous inquiry, involving frequent examinations of the insides of many different living animals and the collation of many observations, I considered that I had achieved my object and got clear from this tangle, while at the same time acquiring exact knowledge about the movement and function of the heart and – in so far as I needed – about the arteries. In consequence I had no hesitation in propounding my view on this matter both in private to friends and in public, College fashion, in my anatomical lectures.

As happens, this view was acceptable to some, to others less so. The latter tore it to pieces, misrepresented it, and found cause of offence in my departure from the rules and belief of anatomists as a whole. The former asked for fuller explanation of the novelty, asserting that it would be worth investigating and would prove of extreme practical importance. At length I reacted to the entreaties of friends that they should all share in my labours, and also in part to the ill-will of the others who, receiving my statements with biased minds and imperfectly understanding them, kept trying to make a public laughing-stock of me. In consequence, I have been forced to publish these things in print so that all may pass judgment upon me and upon the matter in question. I have, however, done so the more gladly in that Girolamo Fabrizzi d'Acquapendente, after having dealt carefully and learnedly in a special treatise with almost all the parts of animals, left only the heart untouched. Finally, I have published so that, if something useful and serviceable should accrue to the republic of letters through my work in this field, it might perhaps be acknowledged that I have done rightly; also that others might see that I have not lived idly; and that the words of the old man in the comedy,

> No life so perfect ever but that circumstance,
> Increase of years, experience, can changes bring;
> Your so-thought knowledge be but ignorance; those things
> That you believed the finest fail to pass the test,

may perchance prove true now in respect of the heart's movement; or at least that others, given this lead, and relying on more productive talents, may find an opportunity to carry out the task more accurately and to investigate more skilfully.

CHAPTER TWO

The nature of the heart's movement, gauged from dissection of living animals

In the first place, then, in the hearts of all animals still surviving after the chest has been opened and the capsule immediately investing the heart has been divided, one can see the heart alternating between movement and rest, moving at one time and devoid of movement at another. These features are more obvious in the hearts of cold animals, such as toad, serpents, frogs, snails, lobsters, shell-fish, prawns, and all small fishes. They likewise all become more obvious in the hearts of warmer animals, such as the dog and the pig, if you watch them carefully until the heart begins to flag and move more languidly and, so to speak, cease to live. Then indeed will you be able openly and clearly to see its movements becoming slower and less frequent and the pauses longer; and you can inspect and determine more conveniently the nature of the movement and the manner of its origin. At rest, as in death, the heart lies relaxed, flaccid, and weak, and so to speak fallen in on itself.

In respect of its movement and of the time of that movement, three major points are to be noticed:

I. That the heart rises and lifts itself up into a point in such a fashion that its pulsation can impinge on the chest at that time and be felt outside it.

II. Hence it appears to contract but in cross-section rather than the opposite, and to become smaller, relatively long, and narrow. If an eel's heart is taken out of its body and placed upon a board or upon the hand, it shows this. The phenomenon is equally apparent in the heart of small fishes, and in those colder animals in which the organ is conical or relatively long.

III. If the heart is grasped by the hand at the time of its movement, it is found to become relatively hard, that hardness arising from the contraction. A parallel is the contraction and greater resistance felt in the tendons at the elbow if one grasps them by the opposite hand as one moves the fingers.

IV. It is, further, to be observed in fishes, and in colder blooded animals such as serpents, frogs, and others, that the heart is whiter in colour at the time of its movement, changing to a deep blood-red when it ceases to move.

From the above points it seemed to me obvious that the movement of the heart was a sort of generalized contraction along the line of the fibres as a whole, and an equally widespread constriction. For in each movement it seems to rise up, gain in strength, diminish in size and harden, and its actual movement seems to resemble that of a muscle contracting in the line of its tendinous and fibrous components. Muscles in active movement gain in strength, contract, change from soft to hard, rise up and thicken; and similarly the heart.

From these observations one can reasonably say that at the time of its movement the heart becomes generally constricted, that its walls thicken, that its ventricles decrease in volume, and that it expels its content of blood. This is sufficiently obvious from the fourth observation for in its contraction, apart from expressing the blood it previously contained, the heart whitens; thereafter in its relaxation and rest, with the re-entry of blood into the ventricle, the purple blood colour returns to the heart. But no one will be able to doubt further after seeing the contained blood escape in spurts at each movement or pulsation during the contraction of a heart which has undergone a penetrating wound of the ventricle.

At one and the same time, therefore, the following events take place, namely, the contraction of the heart, the beat of the apex (felt outside through its striking against the chest), the thickening of the heart walls, and the forcible expulsion of the contained blood by the constriction of the ventricles.

Thus the exact opposite to the commonly accepted views is seen. The general belief is that the ventricles are being distended and the heart being filled with blood at the time when the apex is striking the chest and one can feel its beat from outside. The contrary is, however, correct, namely, that the heart empties during its contraction. Hence the heart movement which is commonly thought to be its diastole is in fact its systole. And likewise its essential movement is not diastole but systole; and the heart does not gain in strength in diastole but in systole – then indeed is when it contracts, moves, and becomes stronger.

One must also reject completely the idea (though the parallel drawn by the immortal Vesal – of the osier circle and the rushes joined together in pyramid shape – appears to support it) that the heart moves solely in the direction of its straight fibres; that thus, while the apex approaches the base, the sides of the heart bend outwards and the cavities dilate, and the ventricles acquire the shape of a cupping vessel and suck in blood (for the heart contracts and constricts simultaneously along all its fibre-directions). On the contrary, one has to believe that it is the walls and solid part of the heart rather than the ventricular cavities which thicken and widen; and that while the fibres contract from the conus to the base, drawing the former towards the latter, the sides of the heart do not bend outwards into a spherical shape, but rather the opposite, so that every circularly disposed fibre tends to become straighter while it contracts. And, as all muscle fibres, while contracting, also shorten in length, they widen and become thicker along the sides of the heart just as they do in the bellies of [ordinary] muscles. Further, the ventricles narrow, in the heart's movement, not only by the straightening and thickening of their walls, but in addition because, when those fibres (or small muscles containing only straight fibres – all in the wall are circular ones) which Aristotle called tendons (they are different in the ventricles of the heart of the larger animals), contract simultaneously, by a wonderful provision all the internal surfaces of the heart's walls are drawn together in succession, as if lassoed, to produce a more forcible expulsion of the blood content.

Also untrue is the common belief that the heart draws any blood into the ventricles by any movement of its own or by its distension. For the expulsion phase is that of contractile movement; the reception phase is that of relaxation and collapse, the manner of which will become apparent later.

CHAPTER THREE

The nature of the movement of the arteries, gauged from dissection of living animals

In extension of the story of the heart's movement, the following points relating to the movements and pulsations of the arteries need to be noted:

I. At the time when the heart is becoming tensed and contracting, and the chest is being struck, and in short systole is occurring, the arteries are being dilated and producing a pulsation and are in their diastole. Similarly, at the time when the right ventricle is contracting and expelling its content of blood, the artery-like vein is pulsating and being dilated, synchronously with the other arteries of the body.

II. When the left ventricle ceases to move, to pulsate and to contract, the arterial pulsation ceases; indeed even before this, when the ventricle is tensing more feebly, the pulse is scarcely perceptible in the arteries. Similarly, with the right ventricle ceasing its activity, in the artery-like vein.

III. Further, if an artery is cut or punctured, the blood is forcibly expelled from the wound during the actual tensing of the left ventricle. Similarly, if the artery-like vein is cut, you will see the blood burst forcibly from it at the same time as the right ventricle tenses and contracts.

Similarly also in fishes, if the vessel leading from the heart to the gills is cut, you will see the blood forcibly extruded from it at the same time as the heart tenses and contracts.

Similarly, to conclude this list, while in every cutting of an artery the blood gets out by leaping forward for a greater or a lesser distance, you will find that the leap occurs in arterial diastole and when the heart is striking the chest; this is precisely when the organ in question is tensing and contracting, and is in its systole and state of erection; by the same movement also the blood is expelled from it.

From these facts it appears, contrary to common beliefs, that arterial diastole is synchronous with cardiac systole, and that the arteries fill up and increase in volume because blood is forcibly driven into them by the contraction of the heart's ventricles; nay further, that the arteries increase in volume because they are filled up like leather bottles or a bladder, and do not fill up because they increase in volume like bellows. There is just the one cause of arterial pulsation throughout the body, and that is the contraction of the left ventricle; the pulsation of the artery-like vein is similarly related to the contraction of the right ventricle.

An idea of this generalized pulsation of the arteries consequent upon expulsion of blood into them from the left ventricle can be given by blowing into a glove, and producing simultaneous increase in volume of all its fingers. For equally, in correspondence with the tension of the heart, the arterial pulsations become larger, more forcible, frequent, rapid, while preserving the rhythm, volume, and order of the heart beat. Nor should one anticipate, on account of the blood's movement, the intervention of a delay between the cardiac contraction and the dilatation of the arteries (especially of the more remote ones) to prevent their simultaneous occurrence. For the condition parallels that during the inflation of a glove or of a bladder, namely, that through a plenum or an occupied space (for instance, through a drum, and in lengths of timber) a blow at one end occurs synchronously with movement at the other, and, as Aristotle says,[1] 'the blood of all animals throbs within their veins [that is to say, arteries], and exhibits a general pulsatile movement throughout them.' 'Thus', as he says elsewhere,[2] 'the veins pulsate as a whole synchronously and successively inasmuch as they all depend on the heart. It keeps moving, hence so do they. They also indulge in a succession of beats when it does.' We have to note, with Galen, that the early philosophers used the term 'veins' where we use the term 'arteries'.

I happened once to see and to have on my hands a particular case which very clearly established this truth in so far as I was concerned. A certain person had a huge pulsating tumour, called an aneurysm, on the right side of his neck near the point at which the subclavian artery turns down towards the axillae. It had developed through the erosion of the artery itself, and kept

[1]Anim. iii, cap. 9.
[2]De respir. cap. 20.

increasing very greatly in size each day as blood for its distension left the artery in successive pulsations. This was discovered when the body was dissected after death; in life, the right brachial pulse had been very small because the greater part of the blood inflow had been diverted into the tumour and had thereby been removed from its normal course.

We can, therefore, say that, wherever the movement of blood through the arteries is hindered by compression, infarction, or interception, there the more distal arteries pulsate less. For the pulse of the arteries is nothing save the impulse of the blood entering those vessels.

CHAPTER FOUR

The nature of the movement of the heart and of the auricles,
gauged from dissection of living animals

Apart from the points already mentioned it is necessary, in connection with the heart's movement, to make some observations concerning the function of the auricles.

Caspar Bauhin and Jean Riolan, learned men and very skilful anatomists, recall their observations[1] that, if you watch the heart's movement carefully during the vivisection of any animal, you will see four spatially and temporally distinct movements, two of which are proper to the auricles and two to the ventricles. While the views of such eminent men command respect, there are in fact four movements which are distinct in respect of place, but not of time. For the two auricles move synchronously and so do the two ventricles, with the result that there are four movements distinct in respect of place but paired in respect of time. And that happens as follows:

There are, so to speak two synchronized movements, one being that of the two auricles, and the other that of the two ventricles or the heart proper. These two movements are by no means simultaneous, but that of the auricles precedes and that of the heart follows, and the movement is seen to begin from the auricles and to pass on to the ventricles. With everything becoming more sluggish as the heart lies dying, and also in fishes and the colder blooded animals, these two movements become separated by an interval of inactivity so that an apparently revived heart appears to respond to the [auricular] movement, at first relatively quickly and later relatively slowly. Finally, as it sinks to death, it ceases to reply with a proper movement at all, and just gives – so to speak – a slight nod with its head, moving so imperceptibly that it appears to exhibit merely a token movement to the pulsating auricle. In this way the heart ceases to beat before the auricles, so that the auricles may be said to outlive it. The left ventricle is the first of all

[1]Bauhin. lib. ii, cap. 21. Riolan. lib. viii, cap. I.

to stop beating; then the left auricle; next the right ventricle; lastly (as Galen indeed noticed), with all the other parts inactive and dead, the right auricle goes on beating, so that life appears to linger longest in this auricle. And while the heart is slowly dying, one can sometimes see it – so to speak – arouse itself and, in reply to two or three auricular beats, produce a single ventricular one slowly and reluctantly and with an effort.

It is, however, specially noteworthy that, after the heart has ceased to beat but while the auricle is still continuing such activity, a finger placed over the ventricle of the heart still feels the individual [auricular] pulsations in the ventricles. The mechanism is the same as that which we mentioned earlier for the perception of ventricular pulsations in the arteries, namely, the distention caused by the impulse of the entering blood. And, if at this time, with the auricle alone beating, you cut off the apex of the heart with a pair of scissors, you will see the blood flow out from the wound with each beat of the auricle. You will thus realize that the blood gets into the ventricles not through any pull exerted by the distended heart, but through the driving force exerted by the beat of the auricles.

It is to be noted throughout that all that I call beats or pulsations, both in the auricles and in the heart itself, are contractions. First you will clearly see the contraction of the auricles and then that of the heart itself. The auricles can be seen to get whiter as they move and pulsate, especially where their blood content is low (they fill up to form a blood store or blood pool through the natural movement of the blood towards them and the centrepetal force exerted upon it by the movement of the veins); indeed, at their terminations and extremities it is particularly obvious that this whitening is due to their contraction.

In fishes and frogs and similar animals which have a single cardiac ventricle, and for an auricle a sort of bladder very full of blood at the base of the heart, you will very readily see first the contraction of this bladder, and thereafter the corresponding movement of the heart.

But I think it right also to describe here observations which I have made and which disagree with those already detailed. The heart of the eel, and of certain fishes, and even of [domestic] animals, after removal from the body, beats in the absence of its auricles. Nay, if you cut it in pieces, you will see its divisions separately contracting and relaxing so that in them, after cessation of the movement of the auricles, the body of the heart continues to pulsate and to throb. But maybe this is peculiar to those animals which cling more to life, whose essential moisture is stickier, or fattier and more sluggish, and not so readily soluble [in water]. This property is also apparent in eels' flesh, which goes on moving after being skinned, disembowelled, and cut into pieces.

In an experiment carried out upon a dove, after the heart had completely stopped moving and thereafter even the auricles had followed suit, I spent some time with my finger, moistened with saliva and warm, applied over the heart. When it had, by means of this fomentation, recovered – so to speak – its power to live, I saw the heart and its auricles move, and contract and relax, and – so to speak – be recalled from death to life.

But I have also from time to time noticed that, after the heart proper and even its right auricle were ceasing to beat and appeared on the point of death, an obscure movement/undulation/palpitation had clearly continued in the right auricular blood itself, doubtless for as long as this blood was visibly imbued with warmth and spirit.

Something of the sort is very obviously seen in the chicken's egg at the beginning of its development and within seven days from its incubation. First before all other things to appear in it is a drop of blood which throbs (as already noted by Aristotle) and from which, after it has enlarged and after the chick has in part been formed, the auricles of the heart develop; the beats within them bear witness to the continuity of life. When after the lapse of a few days the outline of the body has begun to appear, the body of the heart also develops. For some time, like the rest of the body, it appears whitish and bloodless, and is devoid of pulsation or movement. Indeed, in a human foetus about the beginning of the third month I similarly saw a heart that was formed, but whitish and bloodless. The blood in its auricles, however, was very copious and rich in colour. In the egg, with the embryo enlarged and attaining definitive shape, the heart also enlarges and acquires ventricles by means of which it begins to receive and to transmit the blood.

So that, if anyone wished to look more deeply into the matter, he will not style the heart the 'first to live' and 'last to die'. Instead he will say that the auricles (and the part which acts as an auricle in serpents, fishes and suchlike animals) are alive before the heart proper, and die after it.

Indeed, one may wonder if the blood or spirit earlier has that obscure throbbing within it which I thought it continued to have after death, and if we may say that life begins with that throbbing. Since the sperm of all animals (as Aristotle noted) and the prolific spirit leaves the body with a throb like some animal itself departing. So nature in death, with the course as it were ended, retraces her steps (as Aristotle says[2]) and betakes herself back from the finish to the starting point. As animal development proceeds from non-animal to animal, from non- entity so to speak to entity, by the same backward steps corruption changes from entity into non-entity. Hence that which appears last in animals fails first, and what appears first fails last.

I have also observed that in almost all animals a heart is present, not only (as Aristotle says) in the larger and blood-containing ones but in the smaller, bloodless ones, the crustacea and certain testacea, such as slugs, snails, mussels, crabs, lobsters, shrimps, and many others; indeed, in wasps, hornets, and flies, with the aid of a lens to distinguish the very small objects, I have at the top of the portion called the 'tail' seen the heart pulsating, and have pointed it out for others to see.

In the bloodless animals, however, the heart beats very slowly and at long intervals and in the manner of other animals' hearts that are a-dying. Its contractions are also deliberate, as can easily be seen in the snail, the heart of which you will discover if you open it towards the top next the part corresponding to the liver — the heart lies deep within the right-sided orifice which appears to open and shut for purposes of ventilation, and to be the outlet for the animal's slime.

There is yet another point to be noted, namely, that in winter and relatively cold seasons of the year some bloodless animals (such as the snail) are devoid of pulsation and seem to live more like plants, as do also the other creatures which for that reason are called 'plant-animals'.

It is further to be noted that all animals with a heart also contain auricles or something analogous to these, and that two auricles are always present with a heart which has two ventricles, though the opposite is not equally true. If, however, you look at the structural development in the chicken's egg, the first thing to be seen, as I have said, is merely a vesicle or auricle or throbbing drop

[2]De motu animalium, cap. 8.

of blood; it is only afterwards, with growth, that the heart becomes apparent. So, in certain animals which make no effort towards the attainment of further perfection, a certain throbbing vesicle alone is present, in the form of a red or white point, as the beginning of life; as happens in bees, wasps, snails, shrimps, lobsters, etcetera.

We have here a very small shrimp (*shrimp* being English for the Low Dutch *garneel*) which is often taken in the sea and in the Thames, and which has a completely transparent body. I have often caught one and put it into water and shown it to some of my closest friends so that we could see with the least possible impediment the movements of that small animal's heart, the outer parts of its body hindering not at all our so-to-speak window-seat view of its heart-beat.

In the hen's egg, at four to five days from incubation, I have demonstrated the first beginning of the chick in the form of a little cloud, after removing the egg-shell and putting the rest into clear warm water. In the middle of this small cloud the throbbing point of blood was so tiny that it disappeared from view on its contraction, to reappear as a red point during its relaxation, and thus between being visible and invisible, or so to speak between existing and not existing, it gave a representation of the heart beat and of the beginning of life.

CHAPTER FIVE

The movement and functional activity of the heart

From these and suchlike observations I believe that the movement of the heart will be found to occur as follows:

First the auricle contracts and in so doing sends its content of blood (of which it has abundance as head of the veins, and as the blood store and reservoir) into the ventricle of the heart. When the ventricle is full, the heart raises itself, forthwith tenses all its fibres, contracts the ventricles, and gives a beat. By this means it ejects at once into the arteries the blood discharged into it by the auricle, the right ventricle doing so into the lungs through the vessel which is called the artery-like vein but is, in fact, in both structure and function and in all else an artery, the left ventricle doing so into the aorta and through the arteries to the whole of the body.

Those two movements, one of the auricles and the other of the ventricles, occur successively but so harmoniously and rhythmically that both [appear to] happen together and only one movement can be seen, especially in warmer animals in rapid movement. This is comparable with what happens in machines in which, with one wheel moving another, all seem to be moving at once. It also recalls that mechanical device fitted to firearms in which, on pressure to a trigger, a flint falls and strikes and advances the steel, a spark is evoked and falls upon the powder, the powder is fired and the flame leaps inside and spreads, and the ball flies out and enters the target; all these movements, because of their rapidity, seeming to happen at once as in the wink of an eye. In swallowing too it is similar. The root of the tongue is raised and the mouth compressed and the food or drink is driven into the fauces, the larynx is closed by its muscles and by the epiglottis, the top of the gullet is raised and opened by its muscles just as a sack is raised for filling and opened out for receiving, and the food or drink taken in is pressed down by the transverse muscles and pulled down by the longer ones. Nevertheless, all those movements, made by diverse and opposite organs in harmonious and orderly fashion, appear, while they are occurring, to effect one movement and to play one rôle which we style 'swallowing'.

It obviously happens thus in the moving rôle played by the heart, which is a sort of swallowing and a transmission of blood from the veins into the arteries. If anyone (with these things in mind) inspects the heart's movement carefully in a vivisection, he will not only see, as I have said, the heart rise up and combine with its auricles in one continuous movement, but he will also note a certain undulation and obscure lateral inclination along the line of the right ventricle, which twists lightly as it carries out this task. When a horse drinks and swallows water, one can see that the swallowing and passage onwards of the water into the stomach occur with successive gullet movements, each one causing a sound and an audible and tangible thrill. In similar fashion, with each of those heart movements there is a transmission of a portion of blood from the veins into the arteries, and during it the occurrence of a pulse which is audible within the chest.

The movement of the heart is thus entirely of this description, and the heart's one rôle is the transmission of the blood and its propulsion, by means of the arteries, to the extremities everywhere. Hence the pulse which we feel in the arteries is nothing but the inthrust of blood into them from the heart.

We must hereafter inquire and deduce from other observations whether the heart, beyond transferring the blood, giving it local movement and distributing it, adds anything else (warmth, spirit, or finish) to it. For the moment let it suffice to have shown adequately that during the heart-beat blood is transmitted and conducted from the veins through the cardiac ventricles into the arteries, and distributed to the whole of the body.

This is in some measure conceded by all and is inferred by them from the heart's structure, and from the mechanical arrangement, site, and action of the valves. But they seem to be groping about in the dark and to have errors of vision, and they put together things which are diverse, discrepant and incoherent, and – as shown earlier – base very many of their statements on guesswork.

The greatest cause of indecision and error in this matter seems to me to have been a single one, namely, the close connection of the heart and the lungs in the human subject. When investigators had seen the artery-like vein, and similarly the vein-like artery, disappear in the lungs, they were very much at a loss to see whence or how the right ventricle distributed blood to the body or the left

ventricle drew blood from the vena cava. Galen's words are
evidence of this, where he inveighs against Erasistratus on the
origin and function of the veins and the concoction of the blood.
'You will answer',[1] he says, 'that it has been arranged so that the
blood is prepared in the liver and thence is transferred to the heart,
where it will later receive the remaining final finish to its proper
form. Which indeed does not seem unreasonable. For no perfect
and great work can suddenly be accomplished at the first attempt,
or acquire all its polish from one instrument. If it is so, show us
another vessel which draws off absolutely perfect blood from the
heart and distributes it, as the arteries do spirit, to the body as a
whole.' Here then is a reasonable view disapproved and discarded
by Galen because (apart from not seeing the path for the transfer)
he could not find a vessel capable of distributing the blood from
the heart to the body as a whole.

If, however, anyone were present to defend Erasistratus or that
view which I myself now espouse (by Galen's own admission, it is
in other respects consonant with reason), and if he had pointed to
the aorta as the dispenser of blood to the body as a whole, what, I
wonder, would the answer of that most ingenious and learned
authority, Galen, be? If he said that the artery dispensed spirits
and not blood, he would certainly confute Erasistratus (who
thought that spirits were merely contained in arteries) but would
meanwhile contradict himself and would unbecomingly deny the
view which he championed so fiercely in his own book in
opposition to the same Erasistratus. He proves by many strong
arguments and demonstrates by experiments that blood, and not
spirit, is the natural content of arteries.

But if the immortal Galen would allow (as he does fairly often
in the same passage) 'that all the arteries of the body arise from the
great artery, and that artery itself from the heart'; if in addition he
would admit 'that blood is naturally contained and carried in all
of these arteries, and that those three sigmoid valves placed at the
opening into the aorta prevent reflux of blood into the heart, and
that nature would never by any means have attached them to this
highly important viscus unless they had shown promise of being
of some very great service'; if – I say – this father of physicians
would allow us all these points and in his very own words (as he
does in the book from which I have quoted) I do not see how he

[1] Galen. de placitis Hippoc. et Plat. 6.

could deny that the great artery is a vessel suitable to dispense blood, that has now reached its absolute perfection, from the heart to the whole of the body. Would he perchance still be undecided, like all his followers up to this day, because on account of the close connection of the heart and lung he does not see the paths through which the blood can be transferred from the veins to the arteries?

This doubt disturbs even the anatomists not a little (as they always find the vein-like artery and the left ventricle of the heart full of thick, clotting, black blood) for they have to say that the blood oozes across from right ventricle to left ventricle through the cardiac septum. This pathway I have earlier disproved. So now a new one must be prepared and opened, the discovery of which would ensure that no difficulty existed to prevent (I believe) anyone from being able readily to allow and admit those things which I earlier proposed (about the pulse of the heart and the arteries, the passage of blood from the veins to the arteries, and the distribution of the blood to the whole of the body through the arteries).

CHAPTER SIX

The ways by which the blood is carried from the vena cava into the arteries, or from the right ventricle of the heart into the left one

Since it is probable that the connection of the heart with the lung in man provided, as I have said, the opportunity for going astray, those persons do wrong who while wishing, as all anatomists commonly do, to describe, demonstrate and study the parts of animals, content themselves with looking inside one animal only, namely, man – and that one dead. In this way they merely attempt a universal syllogism on the basis of a particular proposition (like those who think they can construct a science of politics after exploration of a single form of government, or have a knowledge of agriculture through investigation of the character of a single field).

Were they as experienced in the dissection of [living] animals as they are practised in the anatomy of the dead human subject, this matter which keeps all involved in uncertainty would, in my view, be simply and readily clarified.

First, then, in fishes, which as lungless animals have but one ventricle of the heart, the matter is sufficiently proved by direct evidence. For by mere inspection or by inspection after division of the artery (the blood gushing out of it with each heart-beat), it can be openly and visibly demonstrated (as is generally admitted) that the sac of blood lying at the base of the heart and obviously analogous to an auricle, sends blood into the heart, which thereupon clearly passes it on through a pipe or artery or a structure analogous to an artery.

Next, the same can readily be seen in all animals in which there is just one, or for practical purposes one, ventricle as, for example, in the toad, frog, serpents, and lizards. In these, though they are reputed to be endowed with lungs in some way inasmuch as they are vocal (I have very many observations on the wonderful arrangement of their lungs and other things of that sort but they are irrelevant here), it is nevertheless clear from direct observation that the blood is carried in the same manner from the veins to the arteries by the beat of the heart. The way is patent, revealed, manifest; there is no difficulty in discerning it, no room for uncertainty about it. For in these animals the position is just as it would be in man had the septum of his heart been perforated or removed, or its two ventricles made into one. In that case, I believe, no one would have had any doubt about the way by which the blood had been able to cross from the veins into the arteries.

As in fact the number of animals without lungs exceeds the number of those with them, and as similarly the number of animals with only one ventricle of the heart exceeds the number of those with two ventricles, it is easy to decide that in the majority of animals, for the most part and on the whole, the blood is transmitted by an obvious route from the veins to the arteries through the chamber of the heart.

It has, moreover, been borne in on me that the same very obviously holds good in the embryos of animals that have lungs. In the foetus, as is well known to anatomists, four cardiac vessels (namely, the vena cava, the artery-like vein, the vein-like artery, and the aorta or great artery) are united otherwise than they are in the adult.

The first contact and union is that of the vena cava with the vein-like artery. This takes place a little above the point where the cava emerges from the liver, and before it opens into the right ventricle, or gives off the coronary vein. The union results in a lateral anastomosis, that is, a large free opening, oval in shape, perforating from the cava into the artery in question. The opening is unimpeded, hence blood can pass very freely and abundantly through it (as through a single vessel) from the vena cava into the vein-like artery and the left auricle of the heart, and thence into the left ventricle. Further, there is in that oval opening, on the side facing the vein-like artery, a thin but strong membrane, like a lid, which is larger than the opening. Later on, in the adult, the membrane covers over the whole of this opening and, fusing with it at all points, renders it quite impervious and well-nigh effaces it. To revert, however, to the foetus – this membrane is so arranged that, in falling back loosely on itself, it moves easily in the direction of the lungs and the heart, and yields to the blood flowing against it from the cava but, on the other hand, prevents reflux of blood into that vessel. Hence, one may justifiably consider that in the embryo the blood must continuously be passing through this opening from the vena cava into the vein-like artery, and thence into the left auricle of the heart. On the other hand, once it has so entered, it can never flow back again.

The other union is of the artery-like vein (which occurs after that vein has left the right ventricle and is dividing into two branches). It is a sort of third trunk added to these two, an artery-like channel, so to speak, leading obliquely from this point to the great artery and perforating into it. Hence, in the dissection of embryos there appear, so to speak, to be two aortae, or two roots of the great artery arising from the heart. This channel, in the adult, narrows and dwindles in similar fashion to the foramen. Finally, it dries up internally like the umbilical vein, and ceases to exist.

The artery-like channel in question has no membrane inside it acting as an obstacle to the blood flow in either direction. For there are at the mouth of the artery-like vein (of which, as I have said, the channel in question is an offshoot) three sigmoid valves facing from within outwards. These yield easily to the blood flowing by this route from the right ventricle into the great artery, but completely prevent any reflux at all from the artery or from the lungs into the right ventricle, which they effectively shut off. Hence, in this instance also it is proper to judge that in the embryo there is a continuous transference of blood by this route from the right ventricle into the great artery, during the contractions of the heart.

It is commonly said that these two unions, so large, free and open, have been made solely for the nutrition of the lungs: and that in the adult (though the lungs should now crave nutriment in greater amount because of their heat and movement) they cease to exist and are filled up. This is an objectionable and inconsistent fabrication. Equally false is the statement that in the embryo the heart is at rest, inactive and motionless, and that in consequence Nature was forced to make these passages for the maintenance of the lungs. For one has only to look at an egg on which the hen has been sitting, and at embryos just removed from the uterus, to see quite clearly that the heart moves in them as in the adult, and that Nature is under no such compulsion. I myself have often witnessed this movement, and the great Aristotle[1] also testifies to it: 'The pulsation', he says, 'is evident from the

[1] Libro de spiritu, cap. 4.

very outset in the developing heart, as can be noticed in the dissection of living animals and in the growth of the chick from the egg.' Further, we see these routes (both in man and in other animals) open and free not only up to the time of birth (as anatomists have described) but even for many months after birth, nay in certain animals for a number of years, if not for the whole course of life, e.g. in the goose, snipe, and most birds, and in animals, particularly the smaller ones. It was this, perhaps, that misled Botallo into claiming that he had discovered a new passage for the blood from the vena cava into the left ventricle of the heart, and I confess that my own immediate reaction, on first finding this feature in a fairly large adult mouse, was somewhat similar.

These facts make it clear that there is absolute identity between what happens in the human embryo and what happens in others, in which the unions in question are not in the process of abolition. Hence the heart, by its movement, and through very patent pathways, transfers blood very obviously from the vena cava, through both ventricular conduits, into the great artery. The right ventricle receives blood from its auricle and then drives it forward through the artery-like vein and its offshoot (the so-called artery-like channel) into the great artery. The left ventricle, in like manner, simultaneously receives blood (that has been directed from the vena cava, by a different route, through the oval opening) by means of the auricular movement, and by its tension and constriction it drives this blood through the root of the aorta into the same great artery.

Thus in the embryo, while the lungs are idle and devoid of activity or movement, as though they did not exist, Nature uses the two ventricles of the heart as one for the transmission of the blood. And the condition of the embryo that has lungs, but is not as yet making use of them, is similar to that of the animal that has no lungs at all.

The truth is thus as manifest in the foetus [as it is in the adult animal that has no lungs], namely, that the heart by its beat transfers blood from the vena cava and discharges it into the great artery. This it does by routes as free and open as would exist in man if the intervening septum were removed and the cavities of the two ventricles communicated with one another. Since, then, in the majority of animals at all times, and in all animals at some time, there exist such very wide ways for the passage of blood through the heart, it remains for us to make one or two inquiries.

Either we should ask why in certain animals (as in man), and those warmer and full-grown, we believe no transfer takes place through the lung substance such as Nature earlier effected in the embryo (at the time when the lungs were functionless) through ways which she appeared to have had to produce because of lack of a passage through the lungs. Alternatively, we should ask why it is advantageous that Nature (who always does what is advantageous) has in adolescents completely closed to the passage of blood those widely open ways which she previously used in the embryo and foetus, and which she does [continuously] use in all other animals; why she has opened up no other ways for such passage of blood, but has in this manner produced a general hindrance to it.

The matter has thus got to the point that those who ask for the ways whereby in man the blood goes from the vena cava to the left ventricle and the vein-like artery would find it more rewarding and think it more satisfactory (supposing they wished to discover the truth from dissections of living animals) to inquire why in the larger and more perfect animals, and full-grown ones at that, Nature should prefer the blood to be filtered through the lung parenchyma rather than, as in all other animals, through very wide ways (they would realize that these were the only alternative pathways). The answer may be as follows, or at least lie along some such lines. The larger and more perfect animals are naturally warmer and, when full-grown, can reasonably be described as over-heated and hard put to it to get rid of the excess. So the hot blood is carried to and through the lungs to be tempered by the inspired air and to be freed from bubbling to excess. But to settle these points and to give a full explanation is merely to explore the purpose of the lungs' fabrication. It is true that by very numerous observations I have discovered much about these organs and their function and movement, about ventilation as a whole, the need for and function of the air, the remaining kindred matters, and the various different organs produced in animals for this end. Nevertheless, lest I be thought to depart too greatly at this point from my main theme (the movement and function of the heart), and thereby to digress, leave my post, and confuse and evade the issue, I will leave these matters for more suitable exposition later in a special treatise. Those things which remain, to revert to my proposed object, I shall continue to establish.

I maintain that in the more perfect and warmer animals, and full-grown ones at that (as in man), the blood definitely permeates from the right ventricle of the heart through the artery-like vein into the lungs, thence through the vein-like artery into the left auricle, thence again into the left ventricle of the heart. I maintain, firstly, that this can happen; secondly, that it has so happened.

CHAPTER SEVEN

The blood permeates from the right ventricle of the heart through the parenchyma of the lungs into the vein-like artery and the left ventricle

We may agree that this can happen and that there is nothing to prevent it from happening when we think how water, permeating through the earth's substance, gives rise to streams and springs; or observe how sweats pass through the skin, or urine through the parenchyma of the kidneys. It is to be noted in those who use the waters of Spa, or the so-called waters of 'our Lady' in the Paduan countryside, or other waters of a mineral or sulphurous character, or in people who just measure their drink in gallons, that one to two hours suffice for them to pass it all out through the bladder as urine. The digestion of such a quantity must take a little while; and it must flow on through the liver (which all agree produces each day a double flow of juice from the food ingested), the veins, the parenchyma of the kidneys, and the ureters into the bladder.

Whom then do I hear denying that blood, indeed, the whole mass of the blood, permeates through the substance of the lungs just as the juice of the food does through the liver, saying that such cannot happen, and must be regarded as altogether incredible? Such folk (in the words of the poet) allow readily that something can take place when they wish it so, but deny its possibility completely when they do not wish it so. They fear to assert it when it is necessary, and do not fear so when it is unnecessary.

The parenchyma of the liver is denser by far, and that of the kidneys likewise. That of the lungs is of much finer texture, and spongy by comparison with the kidneys and the liver. In the liver there is no inthrust, no driving force; in the lung, the blood is pushed in by the pulsation of the right ventricle of the heart, and by this inthrust the vessels and porosities of the lungs must be distended. Moreover,[1] in breathing the lungs rise

---

[1] Galenus, De usu partium.

and fall, movement that necessitates the opening and closing respectively of the porosities and vessels; as happens in sponges, and in all parts having a spongy-make-up, when they constrict and subsequently dilate. The liver, on the other hand, remaind quiescent and has not been seen to dilate and constrict in this way.

Lastly, everyone agrees that the whole of the juice of the ingesta can pass through the liver into the vena cava in man as in the ox or in very large animals, and people have had to admit exactly this if nutriment is somehow to get through the liver to the veins for the purpose of nutrition and no other way is available. Why, in these circumstances, should they not have equal faith in the same proofs of the passage of blood through the lungs in these post-natal subjects, and assert and believe as did the very skilful and learned anatomist, Colombo, from the size and structure of the vessels of the lungs, and from the fact that the vein-like artery and likewise the ventricle are always full of blood which must have come to them through the veins and by no other path than an intra-pulmonary one? He was, and we are, convinced of the truth of this by what has already been stated, by what has been seen in inspection of living animals, and by other proofs.

Since, however, there are some who defer only to duly adduced authorities, let these men know that this truth can be established from Galen's own words. Indeed, not only can blood pass from the artery-like vein into the vein-like artery and thence into the left ventricle of the heart and afterwards into the arteries, but this happens because of the continuous pulsations of the heart, and of the movement of the lungs in breathing.

There are in the opening into the artery-like vein three sigmoid or crescentic valves which completely prevent blood discharged into the artery-like vein from returning into the heart. That is known to all; indeed, Galen[2] explains the need and function of these valves in the following words. *Throughout,* he says, *there is a mutual intercommunication and opening up of arterio-venous connections, and they exchange blood and spirit through certain invisible and quite narrow passages. Had the entry into the artery-like vein likewise remained patent all the while, and had Nature not found a means of shutting it at need and of re-opening it, the blood could never (in the contracted state of the thorax) have been transferred into the arteries through invisible narrow*

[2] Galen, de usu part., lib. vi, *cap. 10.*

connections. However, neither indrawing nor expulsion are completely simple processes. For, on the one hand, that which is light is more easily drawn in than that which is heavier when the means of access are dilated, and more easily expressed when they are contracted. On the other hand, a wide passage is more conducive than a narrow one to swift indrawing and subsequent expulsion. When the thorax contracts, the vein- like arteries in the lung, pushed and pressed in upon from all sides, express indeed their contained spirit, but also take up through those delicate connections that have been mentioned a certain portion of the blood. This could certainly never have happened had the blood been able to move back towards the heart through a large opening, such as that of the artery-like vein. As it is, with the return through the large opening shut off, it distils off a small amount into the arteries through the small openings that have been mentioned. And in a closely following chapter he says: *The more the thorax contracts increasingly strongly in squeezing out the blood, the more the membranes (i.e. the sigmoid valves) occlude with ever greater precision the opening itself, and permit of no backflow.* Just before this in the same Chapter Ten he says: *Without the valves, a triple inconvenience would ensue. The blood itself would keep travelling over this long course to no purpose, flowing forwards it is true in the diastoles of the lung and refilling all the veins within the organ, but in its systoles, like a sea-tide patterned on Euripus, continually reversing the movement to all parts, which would in no way suit the blood. In itself this may appear of little moment, but the fact that meanwhile it upsets the object of respiration itself can certainly not be regarded as trifling,* and so forth. And a little later he adds: *And still a third inconvenience would have ensued, and that by no means an insignificant one, for the blood would have gone backwards in the acts of expiration, had not our Creator devised that outgrowth of membranes.* This leads on to his conclusion in the Eleventh Chapter. *The common purpose of them all* (i.e. of the valves) *is to prevent things from moving backwards again. But each kind has its own special purpose. In the cases of those which direct things out of the heart it is to prevent backflow into that organ; in the cases of those which direct things into the heart, it is to prevent any outflow from it. For Nature did not wish the heart to be tired by unnecessary work, such as on occasion distributing to a part from which it has been preferable to receive, or frequently withdrawing from another part which should have been receiving. As there are altogether four openings, two in each ventricle, one of each pair leads in and the other out.* And a little later he adds: *Further, since there is one vessel, consisting of a single coat, inserted into the heart, and another, consisting of two coats, extending away from it, a place common to both* (Galen had in mind the right ventricle, but the present writer finds the left ventricle equally indicated) *had to be prepared to serve as a kind of pool to which both belong, but into which blood is carried by one vessel and from which it is dispatched by the other.*

The proof which Galen adduces for the passage of blood from the vena cava through the right ventricle and into the lungs can more rightly be used, if only the names are changed, for the passage of blood from the veins through the heart into the arteries, and I should like so to use it. Thus extracts from the writings of Galen, the revered Sire of Physicians, clearly show the blood passes from the artery-like vein through the lungs and into the small branches of the vein-like artery because of the pulsation of the heart and the movement of the lungs and thorax. They show, further, that the heart is constantly receiving and discharging blood, with the ventricles acting as pools, and that for this reason, of the four kinds of valve present, two subserve entry and two exit of blood. This ensures that the blood does not follow Euripus and become unduly disturbed, moving hither and thither or even backwards to the spot which it should have left, and flowing away from the part to which it should have been directed. In this way the heart would become tired by useless work, and the respiration of the lungs would be impeded.[3] Finally, there is support for our claim that blood is continuously and unceasingly passing through the porosities of the lungs from the right to the left ventricle, from the vena cava into the aorta. For, as blood is continuously discharged from the right ventricle into the lungs through the artery-like vein, and is likewise continuously drawn from the lungs into the left ventricle (as is clear from what has been said, and from the position of the valves), it must continuously make the complete circuit.

In like manner, as blood is always continuously entering the right ventricle of the heart, and continuously emerging from the left one (as reason and sense alike show it to be), it cannot do other than pass right through from the vena cava into the aorta.

[3] See the Commentary of the learned Hofmann on Galen, De usu partium, *lib.* 6. *I saw this book after writing these passages.*

Thus that which dissection establishes as occurring through very wide passages in the majority of animals, and certainly in all animals before they are fully developed, is equally well established as occurring (according to Galen's statements and to what I have said above) in these fully developed animals through the invisible porosities of their lungs and the minute connections of the lung vessels. From which it is clear that one ventricle of the heart (namely, the left one) would suffice to distribute the blood through the body and to withdraw it from the vena cava (which indeed is the way it happens in all lungless creatures). When, however, Nature wished the blood to be filtered through lungs, she was forced to make the extra provision of a right ventricle so that its pulsation would drive the blood through these very lungs from the vena cava to the region of the left ventricle. Thus one has to regard the right ventricle as having been made for the sake of the lungs and the transfer of blood, and not merely for nutrition. It is altogether incongruous to suppose that the lungs need for their nourishment so large a supply of food, so pulsatorily delivered, and also so much purer and more spirituous (as being supplied direct from the ventricles of the heart). For they cannot need such more than does the extremely pure substance of the brain, or the very fine and ineffable fabric of the eyes, or the flesh of the heart itself (which is more directly nourished through the coronary artery).

CHAPTER EIGHT

The amount of blood crossing through the heart from the veins into the arteries; the circular movement of the blood

Thus far I have written about the transfer of blood from the veins into the arteries, the paths through which such crossing is effected, and the manner in which the blood is transmitted and distributed as a result of the heart's pulsation. In respect of which matters there are perhaps some who, after my recalling of Galen's authoritative statements or the reasonings of Colombo or of others, may say that they are in agreement with me. The remaining matters, however (namely, the amount and source of the blood which so crosses through from the veins into the arteries), though well worthy of consideration, are so novel and hitherto unmentioned that, in speaking of them, I not only fear that I may suffer from the ill-will of a few, but dread lest all men turn against me. To such an extent is it virtually second nature for all to follow accepted usage and teaching which, since its first implanting, has become deep-rooted; to such extent are men swayed by a pardonable respect for the ancient authors. However, the die has now been cast, and my hope lies in the love of truth and the clear-sightedness of the trained mind. Now, as to the quantity[1] there was, I thought particularly long and hard about the results of my experimental animal dissections and opening the veins, an enquiry that took various forms; about the symmetry and size of the ventricles of the heart and of the vessels which enter and leave them (since Nature, who does nothing in vain, would not purposelessly have given these vessels such relatively large size), and also about the elegant and carefully contrived valves and fibres and other structural artistry of the heart; and many other points: and when I meditated even further on the amount, i.e. of transmitted blood, and the very short time it took for its transfer, and I also noticed that the juice of the ingested food could not supply this amount without our having the veins, on the

---

[1] On the translation of this passage, please refer to the Introduction, p. xi.

one hand, completely emptied and the arteries, on the other hand, brought to bursting through excessive inthrust of blood, unless the blood somehow flowed back again from the arteries into the veins and returned to the right ventricle of the heart; I then began to wonder whether it had a movement, as it were, in a circle. This I afterwards found to be true and that the pulsation of the left ventricle of the heart forces the blood out of it and propels it through the arteries into all parts of the body's system in exactly the same way as the pulsation of the right ventricle forces the blood out of that chamber and propels it through the artery-like vein into the lungs; finding, further, that the blood flows back again through the veins and the vena cava and right up to the right auricle in exactly the same way as it flows back from the lungs through the so-called vein-like artery to the left ventricle (as already described).

We have as much right to call this movement of the blood circular as Aristotle had to say that the air and rain emulate the circular movement of the heavenly bodies. The moist earth, he wrote, is warmed by the sun and gives off vapours which condense as they are carried up aloft and in their condensed form fall again as rain and re-moisten the earth, so producing successions of fresh life from it. In similar fashion the circular movement of the sun, that is to say, its approach and recession, give rise to storms and atmospheric phenomena.

It may very well happen thus in the body with the movement of the blood. All parts may be nourished, warmed, and activated by the hotter, perfect, vaporous, spirituous and, so to speak, nutritious blood. On the other hand, in parts the blood may be cooled, coagulated, and be figuratively worn out. From such parts it returns to its starting-point, namely, the heart, as if to its source or to the centre of the body's economy, to be restored to its erstwhile state of perfection. Therein, by the natural, powerful, fiery heat, a sort of store of life, it is re-liquefied and becomes impregnated with spirits and (if I may so style it) sweetness. From the heart it is redistributed. And all these happenings are dependent upon the pulsatile movement of the heart.

This organ deserves to be styled the starting point of life and the sun of our microcosm just as much as the sun deserves to be styled the heart of the world. For it is by the heart's vigorous beat that the blood is moved, perfected, activated, and protected from injury and coagulation. The heart is the tutelary deity of the body, the basis of life, the source of all things, carrying out its function of nourishing, warming, and activating the body as a whole. But we shall more fittingly speak of these matters when we consider the final cause of this kind of movement.

To conclude, though veins are precise channels and vessels for the carriage of blood, they are of two kinds, the cava and the aorta, not because these lie on opposite sides of the body (Aristotle's view) but by virtue of difference in function, and not (as commonly held) because they are structurally dissimilar (since in many animals, as I have stated above, a vein does not differ from an artery in the thickness of its coat) but because they are distinct from each other in office and usage. Though vein and artery were not unreasonably both styled veins (as Galen noted) by the ancients, one of them, namely, the artery, is a vessel which carries blood from the heart to the component parts of the body, while the other is a vessel which carries blood from those component parts back to the heart. The one is a channel from, the other a channel to, the heart. The latter channel contains cruder, worn-out blood that has been returned unfit for nutrition; the former contains mature, perfected, nutritive blood.

CHAPTER NINE

The existence of a circuit of the blood proved by confirmation of the first supposition

But lest anyone say that we cheat and merely make plausible assertions without a basis and advance new views without just cause, there are three suppositions which come up for confirmation. If these are stated, then I think the truth which I advocate automatically follows and the fact is plain to all.

The first supposition is that the blood is continuously and uninterruptedly transmitted by the beat of the heart from the vena cava into the arteries in such amount that it cannot be supplied from the ingesta, and thus in such wise that the whole mass of the blood passes across from the vena cava into the arteries within a short space of time.

The second supposition is that the blood is continuously, evenly, and uninterruptedly driven by the beat of the arteries into every member and part, entering each in far greater amount than is sufficient for its nutrition or can be supplied to it [without such rapid circular movement] by the whole mass of the blood.

The third supposition, similarly, is that the veins themselves are constantly returning this blood from each and every member to the region of the heart.

With these suppositions thus stated, I think it will be manifest that the blood goes round and is returned, is driven forward and flows back, from the heart to the extremities, and thence back again to the heart, and so executes a sort of circular movement.

Let us estimate, either theoretically or by actual testing, how much blood the left ventricle holds in its dilated state, that is, when it is full. Say this is two or three or one and a half ounces — I have found over two in a cadaver. Let us similarly estimate how much less the heart holds in its contracted state, in other words, what is the degree of its contraction; how much the ventricle's capacity is reduced in its contraction or contractions; how much blood it extrudes into the aorta — that it always extrudes some has been shown in Chapter Three above, and is agreed by all on the evidence of the structure of the valves. From all this let us feel that we may, by a reasonable inference, declare the amount ejected into the artery to be a quarter or a fifth or a sixth, or at the least an eighth, part of the dilated ventricle's content.

In man, then, let us take the amount that is extruded by the individual beats, and that cannot return into the heart because of the barrier set in its way by the valves, as half an ounce, or three drachms, or at least one drachm. In half an hour the heart makes over a thousand beats; indeed, in some individuals, and on occasion, two, three, or four thousand. If you multiply the drachms per beat by the number of beats you will see that in half an hour either a thousand times three drachms or times two drachms, or five hundred ounces, or other such proportionate quantity of blood has been passed through the heart into the arteries, that is, in all cases blood in greater amount than can be found in the whole of the body. Similarly in the sheep or the dog. Let us take it that one scruple passes in a single contraction of the heart; then in half an hour a thousand scruples, or three and a half pounds of blood, do so. In a body of this size, as I have found in the sheep, there is often not more than four pounds of blood.

In the above sort of way, by calculating the amount of blood transmitted [at each heart beat] and by making a count of the beats, let us convince ourselves that the whole amount of the blood mass goes through the heart from the veins to the arteries and similarly makes the pulmonary transit.

Even if this may take more than half an hour or an hour or a day for its accomplishment, it does nevertheless show that the beat of the heart is continuously driving through that organ more blood than the ingested food can supply, or all the veins together at any given time contain.

Nor should it be said that the heart in its contraction varies between extruding a virtual nothing and an imaginary something, such a view having been already confuted, and in addition being contrary to sense and to reason. For, if the ventricles must fill up again with blood in the heart's diastole, they must always extrude blood in their systole, and that in no niggardly fashion (since the blood channels are not small or the degree of the heart's contraction minute), whether the fraction be taken as a third or a sixth or an eighth of the original volume. The ratio of the blood that escapes expulsion to that previously contained in the ventricle and refilling it in its diastole must likewise correspond to that obtaining between the capacity of the ventricle in its contracted state and the capacity of the same chamber in its dilated state. And, as in its dilatation it cannot be refilled with a zero or imaginary charge of blood, so in its contraction it never expels a zero or imaginary amount, but always a positive one proportionate to the degree of that contraction. Whence it is to be concluded that, if the heart in one beat in man, the sheep, or the ox, emits one drachm, and there are a thousand beats in half an hour, ten pounds five ounces have been transmitted in the same time; if in one beat it emits two drachms, the total is twenty pounds ten ounces; if in one beat half an ounce, the total is forty one pounds eight ounces; finally, if it is an ounce at each beat, eighty three pounds four ounces have been transfused in half an hour from the veins into the arteries. But how much is extruded at each heart beat in the individual pulsations, and when more and when less, and for what reason, will perhaps be made clearer by me later as a result of numerous observations.

Meanwhile this much I know, and may I remind all men of it, that the blood makes the passage at times in greater, at times in lesser, amount; and that its circuit is effected now more rapidly and now more slowly according to temperament, age, external and internal causes, things natural and non-natural, sleep, rest, feeding, exercises, mental affections, and the like. But indeed, if the blood passes in even minimal amount through the lungs and the heart, it is carried to the arteries and to the whole of the body in far richer amount than can be supplied from the ingestion of foodstuffs or, in general, without it making a circuitous return.

This we see clearly when we watch the dissection of living animals. For not only when the aorta is opened but also (as Galen establishes in respect of the human subject) if even a very small artery is divided, the whole mass of the blood, within the space of half an hour or less, will be withdrawn from the veins as well as the arteries throughout the body. Butchers, likewise, can produce adequate confirmation of this truth. For, if the neck arteries are cut in the slaughtering of an ox, they drain off the whole mass of the blood, and empty all the vessels, in under a quarter of an hour. In the amputation of limbs or the excision of tumours, I have sometimes found a rapid occurrence of the same end-effect.

The force of this argument is not lessened by allegations that the venous outflow of blood equals or exceeds the arterial one when an animal's throat is cut or human limbs are amputated. For the opposite is in fact what happens. The veins, since they collapse, and have no intrinsic power to force blood out of themselves, and since (as will appear later), the situation of their valves is an obstacle, produce very little blood. The arteries, on the other hand, spout out relatively freely and abundantly a rushing torrent of blood. But you should put the matter to the test in a sheep or a dog by leaving the vein intact and incising the neck artery alone. This will give you a striking impression of the vehemence, force, and rapidity with which the body as a whole loses all its blood, leaving both veins and arteries empty. From what I have said above, it is clear that the blood which the arteries receive can only reach them by being passed through the heart. If, therefore, you ligate the aorta near the root of the heart, and open the neck-artery, or some other one, you will without doubt see nothing but empty arteries and full veins.

From my supposition you will see plainly why, in dissections, so much blood is found in the veins, but little in the arteries; why much in the right ventricle, little in the left one. It was, perhaps, this difference which gave the ancients occasion for doubt and led them to think that, during the life of the animal, spirits alone were contained in those cavities [i.e. in the arteries]. The real reason is, perhaps, that blood can pass from the veins into the arteries in no other way than through the heart itself and the lungs. When these latter have stopped moving at the end of expiration, the blood is prevented from flowing out of the small branches of the artery-like vein into the vein-like artery and thence into the left ventricle of the heart (in the embryo we earlier noted that it had been prevented because the lungs were motionless and so did not open and close successively the minute connections of the vessels and the invisible porosities). As, however, the heart does not cease to move when the lungs do, but continues thereafter to beat and to survive, the left ventricle and the arteries go on discharging blood systematically round the body and into the veins, but receive no replenishments through the lungs and are thus virtually emptied. But even this is some encouragement to belief in my contention, since no other reason can be adduced for the phenomenon save that which I state as deriving from my supposition.

In addition it is clear from the supposition that the more often or more strongly the arteries pulsate, the more rapidly will the body be exhausted of blood in haemorrhages. It is also clear that, whenever the heart beats more languidly, more feebly, and without vigour, any haemorrhage is allayed and held in check.

Further, the supposition explains why in a cadaver, after the heart has stopped beating, you will be unable by any effort you make to withdraw from the opened neck or leg veins and arteries more than a half of the blood mass. Nor will a butcher be able to bleed an ox completely, after stunning it with a blow on the head, unless he has cut its throat before the heart has ceased to beat.

Finally, my supposition allows me to surmise why no one has yet made a correct statement about the site, mechanism, and causation of the anastomosis of the veins and the arteries. I am now busy with that research.

CHAPTER TEN

*The first supposition, about the amount of blood crossing
through the heart from the veins into the arteries, and the
existence of a circuit of the blood, is defended from objections
and is further confirmed by experiments*

So far the first supposition is confirmed by resort to numerical
calculation or by reference to experiments and to observations
which I have myself made, this supposition being that blood is
continuously passing into the arteries in greater amount than can
be supplied from the food ingested, so that, as the whole mass of
the blood passes that way in a short space of time, it must make a
circuit and return to its starting-point.

If, however, anyone objects that a large amount can pass
through without any need for it to make a circuit and that
replenishment from the food intake can occur on a lavish scale, as
is exemplified by the production of milk in the mammae – the
daily yield of a cow is three, four, seven or more gallons and that
of a woman suckling a single child or twins two or three half-pints
per day, and these amounts must clearly be replaced from the food
intake – then the answer should be that the heart, by calculation,
expels this amount or more in one or two hours.

The objector may remain unconvinced and insist on adding
that, although the blood can escape with abnormal rapidity when
an artery is cut open to give it free exit, in the intact body with no
way out provided and with the arteries filled or in their normal
state, so great an amount of blood cannot pass through them in so
short a space of time that it needs must make the return journey to
the heart. To this the answer should be that our previous
reckoning shows, on balance, that the extra amount of blood
contained in the full, dilated heart as compared with that
contained in the constricted heart is for all practical purposes the
amount which is emitted at each heart beat, and so passes in such
quantity into the arteries, in the intact body in its natural state.

In serpents and certain fish, through the ligation of veins a
certain distance from the heart, you will see the rapid emptying of

a stretch of vessel between the ligature and the heart so that, unless you deny the evidence of your own eyes, you must acknowledge that the blood returns to the heart. The same fact will also become clearly evident below in the confirmation of my second supposition.

Let us conclude our confirmation of all these present matters with an example which can convince each and every one through the testimony of his own eyes. If he opens up a live snake, he will for more than a whole hour see the heart beating gently and distinctly, contracting along its length like a worm in its constrictive phase (since it is oblong in shape), expelling its content, in systole becoming paler and in diastole the opposite, and doing practically all the other things which I said were going to provide clear confirmation of this truth for which I contend, for in the snake everything takes relatively longer and is much more distinct. A special experiment which you can make and which is more illuminating than the light of noon is the following. The vena cava goes into the lower part of the heart, the artery leaves from the upper one. If the vena cava is seized with forceps or with the finger and thumb and the course of the blood is interrupted some distance below the heart, you will see at once an almost complete emptying, through the pulsation, of the part between the fingers and the heart, the blood being drawn out of it by that pulsation; at the same time the organ in question is, even in its dilated state, much whiter in colour, and because of its loss of blood smaller in size; in course of time, also, it beats more and more slowly until finally it appears to die. On the other hand, if the vein is released from the pressure upon it, the heart regains its colour and its size. If, after all that, you leave the vein and similarly ligate or compress the arteries some distance away from the heart, you will have the opposite picture and will see the arteries swell up violently between the heart and the constriction, the heart become excessively distended, turn purple to livid in colour, and finally be so oppressed with blood that you believe its suffocation to be imminent. On release of the ligature, however, it reverts to its normal condition in respect of colour, size, and pulsation.

There are, then, two kinds of death: failure from deficiency and suffocation from excess. Here you can see an example of each kind and confirm in the heart with your own eyes, the truth that I have stated.

CHAPTER ELEVEN

The second supposition is confirmed

In order that the second supposition which I have to confirm may be better appreciated by my readers, I must refer to certain experiments which make it clear that the blood goes into each member through the arteries and flows out of it through the veins; that the arteries are the vessels which carry blood away from the heart, and the veins the vessels and pathways for the return of the blood to the same heart; that in the members and extremities the blood passes from the arteries into the veins either directly by anastomosis, or indirectly through the porosities of the flesh, or in both ways, just as it passes (see earlier) from the veins into the arteries in its cardio-pulmonary course. Hence it is manifest that it moves from one region to a second and back again, that is to say, from the centre to the farthest parts and thence back to the centre. If after that premise you make a calculation as before, it will at that very point be manifest that such an amount of blood cannot be supplied from the food intake or necessarily be required for nutrition.

At the same time, a number of points will be manifest in respect of ligatures, the first being the means by which they *draw*, which is not heat, or pain, or suction, or any previously acknowledged cause; the second point, in like manner, the potential convenience and usefulness of ligatures in the practice of medicine; the third, the manner in which they suppress or provoke haemorrhage respectively; the fourth, the reason why they produce gangrenes and mortifications of the members and are thus of use in the castration of certain animals, and in the removal of fleshy tumours and of warts. It is, indeed, because no one has rightly understood the causes and rational basis of all the above that nearly all follow the ancients and propose and counsel ligatures in the treatment of disease, few, however, by the correct use of such appliances adding in any way to the effectiveness of their treatments.

A ligature can be tight or medium tight. I call it the former when the part is so closely compressed by the bandage or noose that no pulsation is perceptible in the arteries anywhere beyond the ligature. Such a ligature we use in the excision of parts when we anticipate haemorrhage. Such, again, they use in the castration of animals and the removal of tumours; it completely interrupts the forward flow of nutriment and of heat, and we see the testicles and huge fleshy tumours decline and die and later drop off. On the other hand, I call a ligature medium tight when it exerts a general pressure upon the part but stops short of causing pain and allows a modicum of pulsation in the artery beyond the constriction. Such an one is of use through its *drawing* power and in blood-letting. Suppose the site chosen for its application is above the elbow, you will be able with your fingers to feel a modicum of pulsation in the arteries at the wrist, provided the ligature is correctly applied in a phlebotomy.

Now make a test on a man's arm by applying such a bandage as they use in blood-letting, or by employing a more than usually strong handgrip. The test is better made in a lean subject with rather wide veins when the body as a whole has become heated and the extremities are in consequence hot, fuller of blood, and pulsating with unwonted force. In such a limb everything will be much more clearly seen.

Thus, if a tight ligature is made by compressing the arm as firmly as is bearable, it can first be noted that beyond the ligature, that is towards the hand, there will be no arterial pulsation in the wrist or anywhere else; secondly, that directly above the ligature the artery commences to be at a higher level in its diastole, and to pulsate more, with greater excursion, and with more force; near the ligature itself it exhibits a kind of tidal swell as if it were trying to burst through an impediment to its passage and to reopen a channel that has become blocked; the artery, moreover, appears abnormally full. Finally, the hand will retain its colour and arrangement; it will just become a little cooler in the course of time, but nothing is *drawn* into it.

After this tight ligature has been on for some time, loosen it suddenly into a medium tight one such as I said they use in blood-letting, and you should see an immediate coloration and disten-tion of the whole hand, with swelling and varicosity of its veins. You will also, in the space of ten or twelve beats of its artery, perceive that the hand has become swollen to bursting by the blood that has been forcibly driven into it; further, that quite a large amount of blood has been *drawn* by this medium tight ligature, and that without pain, or heat, or suction, or any other previously mentioned cause.

If at the exact moment that the ligature is loosened one carefully places a finger near it upon the now pulsating artery, one will feel the blood sliding forward, as it were, underneath it and away. Moreover, the actual subject upon whose arm the test is being made, from the very time that the tight ligature is loosened into a medium tight one, will instantly and clearly feel the warm blood entering at each arterial beat now that, so to speak, the obstacle in its way has been removed. And he will have a sensation along the course of the arteries as if something was suddenly distending them and being dispersed throughout the hand; he will also feel his hand itself becoming warm and tense.

Just as in a tight ligature the arteries above the ligature are distended and pulsate, but not those below it, so – per contra – in a medium tight ligature the veins below the ligature swell up and are resistant, but those above behave quite differently – the arteries diminish in size. Nay, if you compress the swollen veins you must do so strongly if you are to see any great flow of blood or venous distension above the ligature.

So from these facts any reasonably careful observer can readily learn that the blood enters through the arteries, for a tight ligature of those vessels does not *draw* anything; the hand keeps its colour, nothing flows into it, and it is not distended. When, however, the arteries are freed a little (as they are on change to a medium tight ligature), it is clear that the blood is being driven into them forcibly and strongly and in adequate amount, and that the hand is swelling up. Where the arteries pulsate of course, the blood flows on, as it does in the case of a medium tight ligature, in the hand; but where they are pulseless, as in a tight ligature, there is no flow save above that ligature. Meanwhile, there can be no inflow through the veins when these are compressed, and this is indicated by two facts (i) that they are much more swollen below the ligature than they are above it or are wont to be after its removal, and (ii) that when compressed they supply nothing to the parts above. So obviously the ligature prevents the return of blood through the veins to the parts above, and causes the veins below itself to remain swollen.

The arteries, however, find a medium tight ligature no obstacle and naturally enough, through the driving force of the heart, they send blood on from the inner parts of the body to those beyond the ligature. The difference between a tight and a medium tight ligature is that the former interrupts the passage of the blood not only in the veins but also in the arteries, whilst the latter (the medium tight one) does not prevent the pulsatile force from extending beyond the ligature and propelling the blood to the extremities of the body.

It is thus permissible to reason as follows. When we see the veins being rendered turgid and swollen by a medium tight ligature, and the hand getting very full of blood, how does this come about? For the blood must get under the ligature through the veins or through the arteries or through the invisible porosities. It cannot come from the veins and still less can it do so through the invisible channels, so it must come through the arteries in accord with previous statements. It is clear that it cannot flow in through the veins, since it cannot be pressed across to the heart side of the ligature site without complete removal of the actual ligature. When that is done, there is evident a sudden collapse of all the veins as they empty into the parts above, the hand gets whiter, and all the accumulated material, with the swelling and the blood, make a satisfactory disappearance.

Further, the subject who has had his wrist or his arm ligated for an appreciable time past in this way, and whose hands have in consequence become swollen and somewhat cooler – this subject himself, I say, will feel, from the moment the medium tight ligature is taken off, a cold something pass upwards as far as the elbow or the axillae at the same time, presumably, as the blood returns. Such return of cold blood to the heart with release of the bandage after phlebotomy has, I should think, been the reason for the unconsciousness which I have sometimes seen supervene in even strong subjects, especially just after release of the ligature. The common term for the phenomenon is the *turning* of the blood.

Moreover, when through intra-arterial blood flow we see a persistent swelling up of the veins, but not of the arteries, beyond a ligature just after it has been loosened from a tight into a medium tight one, this is a sign both that the blood is flowing from the arteries into the veins (and not in the opposite direction), and also that either there is an anastomosis of vessels or else the porosities of the flesh and solid parts are pervious to blood. A further sign which shows that most of the veins intercommunicate is the fact that in a medium tight ligature, made above the elbow, many of these vessels simultaneously become prominent and swell up; if with a scalpel an exit is made for the blood from but one small vein, all of them at once lose their turgidity and practically all, discharging through that one, simultaneously collapse.

From these facts all can understand the causes of the *drawing* produced by ligatures, and perhaps of fluxion in general; for example, the way in which in the hand the veins are compressed through the action of the sort of ligature which I style medium tight, and the blood cannot get out of them. The consequence is that, when the blood is driven into the hand through the arteries by the force exerted by the heart but is unable to get out again, the part must become full and distended. How otherwise, indeed, can it happen? Warmth and pain and suction *draw*, it is true, but in such fashion that the part merely fills up, and not in such fashion that it becomes distended or swollen beyond the normal limit and, because it is stuffed tight with a forcible inthrust of blood, is so violently and suddenly overwhelmed that the flesh is torn and vessels ruptured. That such can occur through heat or pain or suction is neither credible nor demonstrable.

Further, a ligature can be a *drawing* force without any pain, heat, or suction coming into question. For, if blood could be *drawn* by some pain, how is it that, when the arm is ligated at the elbow, the hand and fingers and veins swell up beyond the ligature and the veins show varicosis (since the compression exerted by the ligature prevents blood from reaching the part through the veins)? And why, above the ligature, can one not see some sign of swelling or fulness or venous turgescence or at least some trace of *drawing* or afflux to the part. But the manifest cause of the *drawing* below the ligature and of the abnormal degree of swelling-up seen in the hand and the fingers, is just that the blood enters in force and in abundance, but is unable to escape.

Can, indeed, the reason for all swelling and overpowering excess in a part simply be (as Avicenna states in respect of swelling) that the ways in are open and the ways out are closed, so that overfilling and swelling-up are inevitable? Is this also the reason why in inflammatory tumours a full pulse is perceptible so long as the swelling is increasing in size but not after it has reached its limit, such being particularly true of swellings which are warmer and show a sudden increase in size? But these are matters for a later discussion. As also is the question whether a certain chance experience of mine can be similarly explained. I once fell from my carriage and struck my forehead on the spot where an arterial branch passes forward from the temples. At once, [that is] in the space of about twenty pulsations from receipt of the blow, I developed a swelling the size of an egg, without either heat or much pain; because, I presume, of the nearness of the artery, blood was being forced into the bruised part in greater abundance and at a greater speed. Moreover, it is clear from my supposition why in phlebotomy, when we wish the blood to spurt farther and more forcibly, we put the ligature on above, and not below, the point where we are to cut. For, had such an amount of blood to flow through the veins from the parts above in order to get out through the opening, the ligature in question would not only not help, but would in fact be a hindrance. The ligature ought more probably to be applied below the opening (to let the retained blood out in greater amount) if the blood, coming down to it through the veins from the parts above, had to escape through the veins. As, however, it is driven from another source through the arteries into the veins below the ligature, while at the same time its return within them past the ligature is prevented, these vessels become turgid and, because of their distension, are able to force the blood out more powerfully through the opening and to eject it farther. When, however, the ligature is loosened and the return route is re-opened, the blood no longer gets out except in drops, and – as all know – if you loosen the bandage in the course of a phlebotomy, or put the ligature below the point of section, or constrict the arm with too tight a ligature, then the blood escapes without force. This is undoubtedly because, in the latter case, the entry and the inflow are interrupted by the tight ligature; and, in the former case, because loosening of the ligature permits a freer return of the blood through the veins.

CHAPTER TWELVE

The existence of a circuit of the blood proved by confirmation of the second supposition

These things being so, it is clear that the other point which I was making above, namely, that the blood is continuously passing through the heart, will also be confirmed. We have seen that the blood crosses over from the arteries into the veins and not from the veins into the arteries. We have also seen that, when a suitable ligature is applied, practically the whole of the blood in the body can be drained off from the area above through an opening made with a scalpel in but a single cutaneous vein. Further, we have seen that the blood escapes so hurriedly and profusely that not only is there a short, speedy evacuation of all that before the cut has been included in the arm below the ligature, but also an extension of this process to the arterial and venous blood content of the arm and of the body as a whole.

Hence it must be conceded, first, that the blood is supplied forcibly and impetuously and is forcibly driven below the ligature (for its escape is forcible and impetuous), the force in question deriving from the pulsatile strength of the heart, which is the sole source of such blood-propulsive power. Secondly, it must similarly be conceded that this flow of blood comes from the heart, and makes its escape by the opening in the arm vein after passing earlier from the great veins through the heart. For it enters the part below the ligature through the arteries and not through the veins, and the arteries nowhere receive blood from the veins save from the left ventricle of the heart; nor, in general, could so great an amount have been withdrawn from one vein with a ligature applied above it – especially so impetuously, abundantly, easily and suddenly – save in consequence, in the way stated, of the forcible cardiac impulse.

And if these things are so, we can also very obviously from my supposition calculate the amount and prove the circular movement of the blood. If, for instance, in a phlebotomy one allowed it to flow out for half an hour with its wonted prodigality and impetuosity, there is no doubt that, after withdrawal of most of the blood, fainting and syncope would ensue, and not only the arteries, but also the great veins would be practically emptied. One can, therefore, reasonably assume that in that space of half an hour such amount of blood has passed from the vena cava into the aorta. Further, if you reckon up how many ounces of blood flow through one arm or are extruded below a medium tight ligature in twenty or thirty pulsations, you will definitely have the means for estimating how much meanwhile passes through the opposite arm, the two legs, the two sides of the neck, and all the other arteries and veins of the body. To all these the flow through the lungs and the ventricles of the heart must furnish ever-fresh supplies of blood, which means that it must return from the veins, since it cannot be supplied from the ingesta and far exceeds what is appropriate for the nutrition of the parts.

I should further note that I have sometimes confirmed this truth while carrying out phlebotomies. For, though you have correctly ligated the arm, and cut the vein duly with the scalpel, making appropriate openings and doing everything in orderly fashion, yet if fear or faintness supervenes (from mental trouble or any other cause) and the heart beats more feebly, the blood will escape in drops only, especially if the ligature has been applied a little more tightly than usual. The reason is that the feebler heart beat and weaker driving force are unable to open the compressed artery and push the blood past the ligature, indeed, the weakened and feeble heart cannot direct the blood through the lungs or transfer it in adequate amount from the veins to the arteries. In the same way and for the same reasons the menstrual fluxes of women, and indeed all kinds of haemorrhage, subside. The opposite pictures also make this clear. For when conditions are restored by return of consciousness and removal of fear, you will see the arteries pulsating again with even greater force in the part that has been ligated, and moving at the wrist, and the blood spurting out again in a continuous jet and farther than before.

CHAPTER THIRTEEN

The third supposition is confirmed; and from it the existence of a circuit of the blood is proved

Thus far I have discussed the amount of blood which passes through the heart and lungs in the centre of the body, and which similarly passes from the arteries to the veins in the peripheral system of the same body. It remains for me to explain how the blood returns through the veins from the extremities to the heart, and how the veins are vessels whose sole function is such carriage of blood back from the extremities to the centre. When I have done that, I think that the three bases for argument which I put forward in favour of the existence of a circuit of the blood will all be evident, true, and irrefutable, and hence will secure adequate credence for my views. The third of my suppositions will be sufficiently evident from the finding of valves in the very lumina of the veins, from the function of these valves, and from ocular demonstrations.

The celebrated Girolamo Fabrizzi d'Acquapendente, a most skilful anatomist and venerable old man, or else (as the learned Riolan would have it) Jacques Dubois, was the first person to depict membranous valves in veins. They consist of sigmoid or crescentic, extremely delicate, raised portions of the inner coat of these vessels, and are separated from one another by intervals which vary from person to person. They arise simultaneously along the vein wall, and look upwards towards the root of the veins and centrally towards the middle of the vein lumen. The twin valves (they occur mostly in pairs) at any one site face, and have contact with, one another; and in the extremities they are so ready to come together and act in unison that they completely prevent any backflow from the root of the veins into the branches, or from the larger into the smaller vessels. They are so placed that the cornua of any one pair of valves face the middle portions of the sinuses of the next pair, and *vice versa*, all the way along the vein.

The discoverer of the valves did not understand their real function, and others went no farther. This function is not to prevent the blood as a whole from rushing down, through its weight, into the parts below. For in the jugular veins the valves face downwards, and here they prevent the blood from moving upwards. In other words, the direction in which the valves as a whole face is not upwards so much as towards the root of the veins and the region of the heart. I, and also others, have sometimes found valves in the renal veins, and in the mesenteric branches facing towards the vena cava and the porta hepatis. A further point is that valves are completely absent from the arteries, and that all dogs and oxen are noteworthy as having valves in the divisions of their leg veins at the commencement of the os sacrum, or in the branches near the hip; vessels in which no such ill effect of the erect stance is to be feared. Nor is it because of the danger of apoplexy, as some allege, that there are valves in the jugular veins; for in sleep matter would be more likely to flow into the head through the sleep-producing arteries. Nor are valves present so that, at points of division of veins, some of the blood may be diverted and brought to a halt in the small branches instead of the whole of it rushing into the more open and more capacious ones. For, even if valves are admittedly more numerous where such points of division occur, they are nevertheless also present in veins which are free from such divisions. Nor is the purpose of valves merely to retard the movement of the blood away from the centre; it is nearer the truth to say that the spontaneous passage of blood from the larger into the smaller branches and thus its separation from its mass and its source, or its passage from warmer regions into colder, is in any case a slow enough one.

No, the sole purpose for which the valves were created was so that the blood should not move from the large veins into the smaller ones (thus rupturing the latter or making them varicose), or from the centre of the body to its extremities, but rather from those extremities to that centre. Hence the delicate valves readily open to allow this latter movement of the blood, but completely suppress the opposite one. They are also so regularly arranged that, if anything is insufficiently held up in its [would-be backward] passage through the horns of the valves above and would, so to speak, slip through the chinks between them, it would be caught up by the transversely placed sinuses of the succeeding valves and be prevented from travelling any farther.

This I very often found in my dissection of veins. If I started from the root of these vessels and tried with all the skill that I could muster to pass a probe in the direction of the small vessels, I was unable to do so over any great distance because of the obstacles provided by the valves; on the other hand, it was very easy to pass a probe from without inwards, that is, from the small branches towards the root of the veins. In the majority of places paired valves are so sited and arranged with relation one to the other that, as they rise away from the vein wall, they come together and meet exactly in the centre of the vein lumen, their free borders being so closely apposed that you could not discern by eye, or adequately trace out, the minute cleft or line of union between them. On the other hand, when the stylet is passed from without inwards, the valves give way even if (like the sluice gates which check the flow of streams) they are very easily turned back again in the opposite direction to check a movement of blood setting out from the heart and the vena cava, and (by their rising away from the vein wall and their mutual apposition in their closure) to bring it to a full stop. They are also so arranged that they nowhere allow the blood to move away from the heart, whether upwards to the head or downwards to the feet or to the sides of the arm. Instead, they resist and oppose all movement of blood which, beginning in the larger veins, ends in the smaller ones, while on the other hand they favour a movement which begins in the narrow veins and ends in the larger ones, and they arrange a free and open channel for it.

But so that this truth may be more openly manifest, let an arm be ligated above the elbow in a living human subject as if for a blood-letting [A A]. At intervals there will appear, especially in country folk and those with varicosis, certain so to speak nodes and swellings [B, C, D, D, E, F], not only where there is a point of division [E F], but even where none such exists [C D]; and those nodes are produced by valves, which show up in this way in the outer part of the hand or of the elbow. If by milking the vein downwards with the thumb or a finger [Fig. 2, O to H] you try to draw blood away from the node or valve [Fig. 2, O], you will see that none can follow your lead because of the complete obstacle provided by the valve; you will also see that the portion of vein [Fig. 2, O H] between the swelling and the drawn-back finger has been blotted out, though the portion above the swelling or valve is fairly distended [Fig. 2, O G]. If you keep the blood thus withdrawn [back to H] and the vein thus emptied, and with your other hand exert a pressure downwards towards the distended upper part of the valves [Fig. 3, K], you will see the blood completely resistant to being forcibly driven beyond the valve [Fig. 3, O]. And the greater the effort you put into your performance, the greater will be the swelling and distension of the vein which you will see at the valve or swelling [Fig. 3, O], though below that the vessel is empty [Fig. 3, H O].

One can find the like at many other points, so the function of the venous valves appears to be the same as that of the three sigmoid valves which have been contrived in the openings into the aorta and the artery-like vein respectively, namely, to close accurately and thus prevent backflow of the passing blood.

Moreover, if, with the arm ligated as before [A A] and the veins swelling up, you press on one of them some distance [Fig. 4, L] below a selected swelling or valve, and thereafter with a finger [M] stroke the blood upwards to the region above the valve [N], you will see that part of the vein remaining empty and the blood unable to pass back through the valve [as in Fig. 2, H O]. When, however, you take your finger [Fig. 2, H] away, you will see the stretch of vein fill up again from the parts below, and become as in Fig. 1, D C. Whence it is clearly established that the blood moves in the veins from the parts below to those above and to the heart, and not in the opposite way. Even if in places valves that do not close as accurately as those mentioned, or are single and unpaired, appear not to present a complete obstacle to movement of blood away from the centre, yet for the most part it is clearly as I have just stated. Or at least something which in one place appears to have been effected with too little care is, it seems, compensated for by the number or competence of the series of valves which follow, or in some other way. So the veins are channels which are widely open to blood which is returning towards the heart but are completely closed to blood moving away from it.

Still another experiment should be noted. In a living human subject, with the arm ligated as before, the veins swelling up and nodes or valves coming into view, select a place where a second valve follows a first, and apply a thumb to occlude the vein and prevent any bloodflow up from the hand. Then with a finger, as detailed above, force the blood up out of that portion of vein [L N] into the stretch above the valve. Now take the finger [L] away and let the vein fill up again from below [as in D C]. Reapply the thumb and again force the blood up out of the vein [Fig. 4, L N, and Fig. 2 or 3, H O], and do this quickly a thousand times. If after that you make a calculation (by multiplying by a thousand your estimate of the amount which is raised above the valve at each upward stroking of the vein), you will find that so much blood passes in a relatively short time through the one portion of vein that, I believe, you will be completely convinced, by the speed of the blood's movement, of the fact that it circulates.

In case, however, you feel like saying that this experiment is unnaturally rigorous, may I suggest that you try it on a vein with widely separated valves, and see how quickly and rapidly, once the thumb is removed, the blood flows upwards and fills the vein from below. I have no doubt that making this test will carry conviction to you.

Figures 1–4 are printed at the beginning of this essay on page 16.

CHAPTER FOURTEEN

Conclusion of my description of the circuit of the blood

May I now be permitted to summarize my view about the circuit of the blood, and to make it generally known!

Since calculations and visual demonstrations have confirmed all my suppositions, to wit, that the blood is passed through the lungs and the heart by the pulsation of the ventricles, is forcibly ejected to all parts of the body, therein steals into the veins and the porosities of the flesh, flows back everywhere through those very veins from the circumference to the centre, from small veins into larger ones, and thence comes at last into the vena cava and to the auricle of the heart; all this, too, in such amount and with so large a flux and reflux – from the heart out to the periphery, and back from the periphery to the heart – that it cannot be supplied from the ingesta, and is also in much greater bulk than would suffice for nutrition.

I am obliged to conclude that in animals the blood is driven round a circuit with an unceasing, circular sort of movement, that this is an activity or function of the heart which it carries out by virtue of its pulsation, and that in sum it constitutes the sole reason for that heart's pulsatile movement.

CHAPTER FIFTEEN

The circuit of the blood is confirmed by probable reasons

It will not, however, be irrelevant to add that, according to certain common reasonings, it should both fittingly and necessarily be thus. First (Aristotle, *De respiratione* and *De partibus animalium*, lib. 2 and 3, and elsewhere), as death is a corruption for lack of warmth and all living things are warm, dying ones cold, there must be a site and source of warmth, a sort of health and home to contain and preserve the natural kindling materials and the beginnings of innate fire, and to act as the source from which warmth and life may flow to all parts and aliment accrue, and upon which digestion, nutrition, and all activity may depend. That this site is the heart, and that the heart is the beginning of life in the way which I have stated, I would have no one doubt.

The blood, therefore, needs movement and that movement such as carries it back to the heart. For if, (as Aristotle says in *De partibus animalium*, lib. 2) it went far away from its source into the outer parts of the body, it would cease moving and clot. In all we see warmth and spirits generated and preserved by movement, but abolished by rest. Hence it was inevitable that the blood, hard-set or frozen by the cold of the extremities and of the environment, and deprived (as in the cadaver) of spirits, should seek from the source and origin a further supply of warmth and of spirits and in general a restoration to health, and by returning to the heart should recruit these.

We see how the extremities are sometimes chilled by the external cold, how the nose and hand and cheeks appear livid like those of dead folk, and the blood in them (like that which is wont to lie in the under parts of cadavers) takes on a leaden-blue colour, and the limbs become so torpid and hard to move that they seem all but dead. They would certainly not (especially so quickly) recover their warmth, colour, and liveliness except they were warmed by the arrival of a fresh supply of heat from the centre. For how can peripheral parts that are cold and all but lifeless attract a fresh inflow? Or how could those with channels packed full of congealed blood admit additional nutriment and blood unless they first rid themselves of that which they already contained? Unless, too, the heart were indeed such a centre as would retain life and warmth with the extremities frozen (see Aristotle, *De respiratione*, Cap. 2), and would transmit through the arteries fresh, warm, spirit-imbued blood to drive out the chilled and effete matter, and to allow the parts to become warm again and revive their all but extinguished vital fire?

Because of this it is possible, provided the heart has remained unaffected, for all the other parts to be restored to life and to recover their health. If, on the other hand, the heart has been chilled or affected by some serious fault, then the whole animal must suffer destruction because its chief organ does so. For there is nothing (Aristotle, *De partibus animalium*, Cap. 3) which this organ can do to help either itself or the rest of the organs which depend upon it. Incidentally, this may be the reason why sadness, love, hatred, and troubles of that kind cause wasting away and thinning, ill humour and multiple indigestions such as introduce all diseases and are killing to men. Every affection of the spirit which stirs human minds with sorrow or joy, hope or anxiety, and extending to the heart changes its natural disposition in respect of temper, pulsation, and the other features: every such affection – I say – pollutes all the ingesta from the outset and weakens the body's powers, so it need scarcely be marvelled at that it often begets various kinds of incurable diseases in the limbs and the body, seeing that the whole body is in that case suffering from vitiation of its food and lack of innate warmth.

Moreover, as all animals live on food which has undergone digestion within themselves, that digestion and the distribution of its products must be perfect. Similarly, there must be a place into which the food in question can be received, in which it can be perfected, and from which it can be distributed to the individual members of the body. This place, you must know, is the heart. For it alone of all the parts contains blood for general use (that is to say, the blood in its auricular and ventricular cavities, which can be regarded as storage cisterns – the other blood, in the coronary vein and artery, is for the heart's private use); all the other parts have blood in their vessels solely for their own ends and for private use. In addition, the heart alone is so sited and arranged that it can, by its pulsation, impartially dispense and distribute blood from itself to all parts according to the relative dimensions of their supply arteries, and thus – so to speak – give freely from its source of wealth to those in need.

Further, for such distributive blood movement, both force and vehemence are necessary and also an agent, such as the heart, to provide such force. In the first place, this is so because the blood tends naturally and readily to move to a concentration point (as a part to the whole, or as a drop of water spilt on a table to the main mass); minor causes such as cold, fear, horror, and the like effect this very rapidly. Secondly, it is so because the blood is expressed, by the movements of the limbs and the compression exerted by the muscles, from capillary veins into venules and thence into comparatively large veins, and is thus more disposed and prone to move centrally than the opposite (even supposing the valves offered no obstacle). So, in order that it may leave its central point and enter narrow and colder parts and go against its inclination, the blood needs both vehemence and an agent to provide it. The only such agent is the heart, and that in the way that I have stated.

CHAPTER SIXTEEN

The circuit of the blood is proved from certain consequences

There are in addition questions, consequent so to speak upon the supposition of this truth, which are not without their use in establishing belief, as it were, *a posteriore*. Though they seem otherwise to be involved in much ambiguity and obscurity, they readily permit the assignation of rational causes from the supposition. Examples of such questions are provided by the things we see happen in contagion, in a poisoned wound, in the bite of serpents or of a mad dog, in venereal disease and the like, the common point being how it comes about that the whole system is vitiated through the relatively harmless touching of but a small part of it. Venereal disease, for example, at times leaves the genitals unharmed, and manifests itself first of all by pain in the scapulae or the head, or by other symptoms; and I have known fever or the other dread symptoms come on after the wound made by the bite of a mad dog has been cured. From the supposition it is clear that the contamination is first imprinted into the part, then reaches the heart in the returning blood, and thereafter from the heart pollutes the whole of the body.

In tertian fever the disease-producing cause, making first for the heart, lingers around that organ and the lungs and brings about shortness of breath, difficulty in breathing, and disinclination for exertion in those affected. For the vital principle is oppressed, and the blood is forced into the lungs, becomes inspissated, and does not get through those organs (I speak with experience on this point through my dissections of subjects who have died at the beginning of attacks). At this time the pulsations are always rapid and small in amplitude, and now and then irregular. However, with increase in [local] warmth, and thinning of the matter in the vessels, the channels opening up and a passage made, the whole body begins to get warmer, the pulsations increase in amplitude and strength, and an increase in the fever as the obviously excessive heat engendered in the heart is passed thence, together with the disease-producing material, through the arteries to the whole of the body. In this way the material in question is overcome by nature and destroyed.

It is also obvious from my supposition why externally applied medicaments exert their powers internally just as if they had been internally taken. Colocynth and aloe loosen the belly, cantharides produce movement of urine, garlic bound to the soles of the feet helps expectoration, cordials give strength, and so on and so on. It is perhaps not unreasonable to say that the veins through their openings absorb a fraction from the substances placed on the outside, and carry it inside together with the blood, just as those in the mesentery suck chyle out of the intestines and carry it together with the blood to the liver.

For indeed in the mesentery the blood enters through the coeliac and superior and inferior mesenteric arteries and proceeds to the intestines; from these, together with the chyle which has been drawn into the veins, it returns through the very numerous branches of those veins into the porta hepatis and, through the liver itself, into the vena cava. For this reason the blood in these veins is of the same colour and consistence as that in the rest of the veins (though this is a minority view), and it is unnecessary to subscribe to the improbable suggestion that in every capillary offshoot there is a two-fold movement, of chyle upwards and of blood downwards. Is the effect not rather due to the extreme ingenuity of Nature? For, if raw chyle were mixed in equal portions with mature blood, the result would not be a maturation, transmutation and sanguification, but rather (as they are respectively active and passive) an intermediary product deriving from the union of the two substances, like sour wine mixture produced by adding water to wine. When, however, a small portion of chyle is mixed with a large amount of passing blood in this way, and it contributes only a small portion of the total mass, the change (as Aristotle says) is effected with comparative ease since, when a drop of water is added to a large jar of wine or *vice versa*, the whole is not a mixture, but is essentially wine or water still. So in opened-up mesenteric veins what is found is not chyme, not chyle and blood, either separate or blended, but sensibly, in respect of colour and consistence, the same blood as in the remainder of the veins. As, however, it contains a modicum, even if an imperceptible one, of chyle that has not undergone concoction, Nature interposed the tortuous hepatic channels to delay the blood and to ensure its more complete transmutation, so that it should not reach the heart prematurely and in imperfect condition, and thereby overwhelm the vital principle. Thus in the embryo the liver is practically functionless, and because of that fact the umbilical vein is seen to pass intact through the organ, an opening or anastomosis leading off from the porta hepatis so that the blood returning from the foetal intestines may pass through the aforesaid umbilical vein rather than through the liver substance and, together with the maternal blood and that returning from the uterine placenta, may make for the heart. This is also the reason why the liver does not appear until relatively late in the developing foetus; indeed, in the human foetus I have seen all the members perfectly delineated, and even the genitalia distinct, at a time when the rudiments of the liver had scarcely been roughed out. And in truth at the time when all the members appear white (like the heart itself at the outset) and, except within their veins, are innocent of any red coloration, you will see at the site of the liver nothing except a shapeless mass of blood which you could take for a bruise of some sort or a ruptured vein.

But in the egg there are, so to speak, twin umbilical vessels, one – from the white part – which passes intact through the liver and tends straight towards the heart, the other – from the yelk – which ends in the vena portae. At the outset the chick in the egg is formed and nourished from the white part only but, after its completion and hatching, from the yellow one. This latter can be found contained within the intestines in the chick's abdomen many days after hatching, and it corresponds with the nutriment supplied by the milk of other animals.

These matters, however, will be more appropriately dealt with in my observations on the formation of the foetus, in which there can be very many questions of this kind. For example, why is this part made or perfected earlier, and that later? And in respect of the relative importance of members, which of two parts is the cause of the other? And several questions about the heart, such as, Why has it been the first (as stated in Aristotle, *De partibus animalium*, lib. 3) to acquire firmness, and why does it seem to have life, movement, and feeling within itself before any of the rest of the body has been perfected? And in like fashion about the blood. Why is it there before all the rest? How does it come to possess the vital and higher principles, and to be eager to move and be driven hither and thither, the object for which the heart appears to have been made? In the same way in observation of the pulsations, Why are particular kinds associated with the imminence of death or the opposite? And in contemplating their origins and prognostics in all types, What do those imply, what that one and why? Similarly in crises and natural cleansing discharges; in nutrition, especially the distribution of food; similarly, too, in all cases of fluxion. When I finally reckon up the number of questions that can be settled, doubts resolved, and obscure places made clear, given this illuminating truth, in every part of medicine (physiology, pathology, semeiotics, therapeutics), I find a field of such vast extent that, if I explored it fully in all directions, not only would this treatise of mine turn, contrary to my plan, into a full-sized book, but the rest of my life would perhaps not suffice for my writing of it.

Here, therefore, that is to say in the next Chapter, I shall merely attempt to relate to their functions and true causes those things which become apparent, in the course of an anatomy, with respect to the structure of the heart and of the arteries. While in every direction that I look I find very many matters illuminated by this truth and in their turn rendering it ever clearer, I wish above all else its confirmation and embellishment by anatomical evidence.

There is one item which should by rights take its place among my observations on the function of the spleen, but to which a passing reference here also will not be irrelevant. From the upper part of the splenic venous branch which comes off in the pancreas, there arise the posterior coronary, gastric and gastro-epiploic veins, all of which, together with their very numerous twigs and ramifications, are distributed to the stomach in just the same way as the mesenteric veins are distributed to the intestines. Similarly from the lower part of that splenic venous branch, the haemorrhoidal vein passes off downwards to the colon and rectum. The blood returning through these two venous systems carries back with it, on the one hand from the stomach a relatively immature juice – watery, thin, and with its chylification not yet perfected, on the other hand a thicker, more earthy juice which can be regarded as deriving from the faeces. In the splenic venous branch there is a thorough mixing of opposites and the blood is suitably tempered. Nature thus deals with the two juices which are resistant, through their respective abnormalities, to coction by mixing them thoroughly and adding to them large amounts of relatively warm blood, supplied in great profusion by the spleen through its multiplicity of arteries. She thus brings the juices to the porta hepatis in a better state of preparation and, thanks to the arrangement of the venous system that I have mentioned, supplements and compensates for what is lacking in both extremes.

CHAPTER SEVENTEEN

*The circuitous movement of the blood is confirmed by things seen
within the heart and revealed by anatomical dissection*

It is not in all animals that I find the heart to be a distinct and
separate part. For some, which you may call plant-animals, are
devoid of hearts as being of too cold a type, too small in body, too
soft in texture, and too little differentiated in their structure. They
include the caterpillars and earthworms and numerous creatures
that arise from decaying matter and have no set appearance. Such
are devoid of a heart as having no need of a propulsive organ to
transmit food to their extremities. For their bodies develop all at
one time as homogeneous, limbless units and in consequence their
intake and expulsion of food is an in and out movement produced
by contraction and relaxation of the body as a whole. The so-
called plant-animals, oysters, mussels, sponges, and indeed
zoophytes of all kinds, are devoid of hearts inasmuch as they use
the whole of the body as such and an animal of this sort is in effect
nothing but a heart. In very many animals, including practically
all the different kinds of insects, the body is too small for us to be
able to distinguish details with certainty. Nevertheless, in bees,
flies, hornets and the like it is possible, if at times the help of a lens
is required, to see a pulsating something within. And even in lice
(in which you will also be able to distinguish, as a sort of black
spot in the otherwise translucent animal, the passage of food
through the intestines) you will perceive the same kind of thing by
using the magnifying glass which I have mentioned.

In some colder animals which are devoid of [red] blood, such as
snails, mussels, shrimps and shell-fish, there is a small pulsating
part, a sort of vesicle or auricle without its ventricle, which
contracts and produces a beat rather infrequently, and can be seen
only in summer or in fairly warm weather. This small part is
present in these animals inasmuch as some driving force is needed
to distribute the blood, either because of the organic variety of the
parts or because of the density of the body's substance. But the
beats occur rather infrequently, as I have already said, and

sometimes, because of the cold, not at all. This is appropriate for creatures of such ambiguous nature that at some times they appear alive, at others dead, at some times to lead the life of an animal, at others that of a plant. This seems also to happen to insects since they disappear in winter and bury themselves as if dead, or else merely continue a plant-like existence. We can, however, reasonably doubt if the same holds good for certain red-blooded animals such as frogs, tortoises, serpents and swallows.

In larger and warmer, inasmuch as red-blooded, animals there is need of an organ to propel the food, and that perhaps with greater force. Hence the provision of both an auricle and a ventricle of the heart in fishes, serpents, lizards, tortoises, frogs, and others of this sort. Whence it is very true to say (Aristotle, *De partibus animalium*, lib. 3) that no red-blooded animal lacks a heart and the food is not only moved on by the auricle, but is extruded to a greater distance and at a greater speed by the stronger and more vigorous propulsive agency of the ventricle. Indeed, in animals that are still larger, warmer, and more perfect as being richly supplied with hotter, spirituous blood in very great amount, a stronger and more fleshy heart is needed to extrude the food more forcibly and quickly and with greater impetus, either on account of the large size of the body or because of the density of its constituents. Further, as the more perfect animals require more perfect food, and a larger supply of innate warmth to concoct that food and make it even more perfect, it was fitting that they should have lungs and also a second ventricle to drive the food through those lungs.

Thus in all animals which have lungs there are two ventricles, a right one and a left one. Also, in any animal in which there is a right ventricle there is also a left one, but the converse does not hold good. I distinguish a left ventricle by function and not by situation; it is, namely, one which distributes the blood to the whole of the body and not to the lungs alone. Thus the left ventricle seems to be the essential part of the heart; it lies centrally, and is engraved with so much deeper furrows and fashioned with so much greater care that the whole heart seems to have been made for the sake of this left ventricle, and the right ventricle to be merely the attendant upon its fellow. This right ventricle does not extend to the apex, its wall is three times as thin as that of the left ventricle, and (as Aristotle says) it has the appearance of being articulated onto its companion; it has, however, the greater capacity inasmuch as it supplies not only material for the left ventricle, but also food for the lungs.

It is, however, to be noted that these matters are otherwise arranged in the embryo, and there is not the same degree of difference between the ventricles, which are arranged almost equally, like twin kernels in a double nut. The cone of the right ventricle reaches to the tip of the left ventricle, so that the heart in the foetus is like a cone with two tips. This is so (as I have already stated) because in the foetus the blood is not passing through the lungs from the right ventricle into the left one. On the contrary, these two chambers are both busy with a single task (namely, the transference of blood from the vena cava into the aorta, though one does it through the foramen ovale, and the other through the artery-like passage, as I have already stated), and have identical parts to play in the propulsion of the blood to the whole of the body. Hence the identity in their dispositions. When, however, it is time for the lungs to function and for the above-mentioned unions to be occluded, the ventricles begin to differ in strength and in the other respects noted, because the right ventricle now propels the blood through the lungs only, but the left ventricle propels it through the whole of the body.

In addition, there are inside the heart numerous small armlets (if I may so style them) of muscle or small twigs of flesh, and fibrous bundles. These structures, called 'nerves' by Aristotle (*De respiratione*, and *De partibus animalium*, lib. 3), in part course separately in a variety of ways, in part are hidden, like a number of small muscles, in furrows that have been deeply cut in the ventricular walls and in the septum between the ventricles. They act as reserves and reinforcements to the heart in its efforts to contract and to propel the blood more strongly and more vigorously, and they assist it in expelling that blood to a greater distance. Like the carefully planned and ingenious arrangement of ropes on a ship, they are intended to assist everywhere as the heart contracts in all directions and to ensure a stronger and more complete expulsion of the blood from the ventricles. This is further clear from the fact that they are present in some animals but scarcely at all in others, and that in all animals in which they are present they are more numerous and more powerful in the left ventricle than in the right one. In some animals they are present in the left ventricle but completely absent from the right one. In man they are more numerous in the left ventricle than in the right one, and in the ventricles than in the auricles; some individuals have practically none in the auricles. They are more numerous in the brawny muscular bodies of country folk and those of relatively solid build, comparatively few in slender subjects and in women.

In those animals in which the inner surface of the heart is smooth (completely devoid of fibres and armlets of muscle) and undivided by furrows (that is, in practically all the smaller birds such as the partridge and domestic fowl, in serpents, frogs, tortoises and the like, and equally in the greater number of fishes), in these animals, I say, no 'nerves' or fibres such as I have just described, and no tricuspid valves, are found in the ventricles. In some animals the right ventricle is smooth inside, but the left ventricle has the fibrous bundles we have been discussing; such animals include the goose and the swan and heavier birds. In these the same reason holds good as in all. The lungs are spongy, loose in texture and soft, and hence less force is required to extrude blood into them. So the right ventricle either has none of the fibres in question, or has fewer or weaker ones which are not so fleshy or muscle-like. Those in the left ventricle, on the other hand, are both stronger and more numerous and more fleshy and muscular because the left ventricle needs greater strength and force to have extended its influence upon the blood throughout the whole of the body. This is also the reason why the left ventricle lies in the middle of the heart and has a wall that is three times as thick and strong as that of the right ventricle. It is, in addition, the reason why all animals (man similarly) have a more fibrous, thicker, stronger and more muscular heart in proportion as their fleshy make-up is denser, harder and more solid, and as their extremities are more fleshy and brawny and farther from the heart. That is both manifest and necessary. On the other hand, the looser their texture and softer their build and lesser their corpulence, the more flaccid, smoother, internally less (or not at all) fibrous, and weak is the heart which they carry inside themselves.

Consider likewise the function of the valves. Those at the entries into the ventricles have been made to prevent the blood from returning once it has been sent into those chambers. Those in the openings into the artery-like vein and the aorta, in ballooning up to meet their fellows, produce a three-cornered line such as is left by the bite of a leech, and this apposition makes for their tighter closure and guards against backflow of the blood. The ventricular valves act as door-keepers in the passages from the vena cava and the vein-like artery into the ventricles, their object being to prevent backsliding of the blood at the moment of its greatest forward propulsion, and for that reason, as I have said earlier, they are not present in all animals. Nor do they appear to have been made with equal skill in all the animals in which they are present. In some they have been made relatively carefully, in others relatively slackly and carelessly, and in consequence the force deriving from the ventricular contraction for their closure varies correspondingly in degree. In the left ventricle, so that the occlusion may be more precise in accordance with the greater force, there are only two mitre-like valves to ensure perfect closure. They pass centrally for a long distance in the direction of the apex, and it was maybe this fact which misled Aristotle, when he had cut this ventricle transversely, into thinking that it was double. To prevent the blood from slipping back into the vein-like artery and thereby reducing the effort of the left ventricle in propelling that blood forwards to the body as a whole, the mitral valves which I have mentioned exceed in size and strength and accuracy of closure the ones situated in the right ventricle. Hence, too, of necessity no heart is seen devoid of a ventricle, since the latter must serve as a chamber for the supply and storage of the blood. The same, however, does not always hold true in respect of the brain, for practically all kinds of birds are devoid of a cerebral ventricle. As is evident in the goose and the swan, the brain in which is scarcely as large as that of a rabbit; moreover, though rabbits have ventricles in their brains, the goose has none. Likewise, wherever there is a single ventricle of the heart, a single auricle in the form of a flaccid, skin-like bag full of blood is appended to it; where there are two ventricles, there are likewise two auricles. On the other hand, an auricle alone, without a ventricle of the heart, is present in some animals, or at least a vesicle analogous to an auricle, or the locally dilated vein itself pulsates, as can be seen in hornets and bees and other insects. That these animals possess not only a pulsatory, but also a respiratory, activity in their so-called tail part, I think I can show by certain experiments. They appear to lengthen and shorten the tail part more or less frequently in accordance with their degree of breathlessness and need for air. But I will say more about this in my treatise on respiration.

It is likewise evident that the auricles pulsate, contract as already stated, and eject the blood into the ventricles. Hence an auricle is required wherever there is a ventricle and not merely, as is commonly believed, to act as a receptacle and storehouse of the blood, for what need is there of a pulsation just in order to retain that fluid? No, the auricles are its initial movers, and this is especially true of the right one, 'the first part to live, the last part to die', as has been stated earlier. It is for this reason that the auricle is needed, that is to say, it has to help to infuse the blood into the ventricle so that the chamber in question may more readily express what has already been set in movement, and may send it on with greater vigour. Just as in a ball-game you will manage to drive the ball harder and farther by hitting it on the rebound than you will by throwing it from rest. Moreover, the general view is wrong, and neither the heart nor any other organ can draw anything into its cavity during its diastole unless it does so as a partially compressed sponge reverting to its original shape; on the contrary, it is axiomatic that all local movement in animals begins in, and originates from, the contraction of some small part. Hence the blood is ejected into the ventricles, as I have already disclosed, by the contraction of the auricles and is projected and carried forward from the ventricles by their own subsequent contraction. This truth about local movement; and the immediate organ of movement which is the contractile element in all movement of all animals in which a spirit of movement (as Aristotle says in *Liber de spiritu* and elsewhere) is primarily present; and the way the word νεῦρον is derived from νεύω, I nod, I contract; and the fact that Aristotle knew about muscles and did not haphazardly refer all movement in animals to the nerves or the contractile element, and hence called those armlets of muscle in the heart by the name 'nerves' – all this would, I should imagine, become clear were I at some time or other allowed to give a demonstration from my observations about the organs of movement of animals and about the functional anatomy of their muscles.

To revert, however, to the function of the auricles in filling the ventricles as pointed out above, it is of interest that the denser, more compact, and thicker-walled is the heart, the more vigorous and more muscular are the auricles for the forward movement of the blood and the filling of the ventricles. In those animals, on the other hand, in which the opposite holds good, the auricle resembles a blood-coloured bladder or a membranous bag of blood, as it does for instance in fishes. In such, this bladder which takes the place of an auricle is so extremely thin and withal large that the heart seems to be floating on top of it; further, in those fishes in which the bladder in question is a little fleshier, it gives a very pretty if misleading impression of lungs, as for instance in the carp and barbel, tench, and others.

In a number of human subjects distinguished for their brawn and toughness of build, I have found the right auricle so strong, and with so complex an internal arrangement of muscle 'armlets' and interlacing fibres, that it appeared to me to equal in strength the ventricles of other subjects, and I was frankly amazed that there could be so much difference between individuals. It must, however, be noted that in the foetus the auricles are relatively far longer because they are already present, as shown earlier, before the heart comes into being or discharges its function, and they deputize for it. Even so, it is my actual observations on the formation of the foetus (as described above, and as confirmed by Aristotle in respect of the egg) which are the most convincing and illuminating contributions about the point under discussion. While the foetus is still like a soft worm or, as the phrase goes, in the milk, all that is visible within it is a bloody point or pulsating vesicle and what appears to be a portion, dilated at its beginning or base, of the umbilical vein. Later on, when the foetus has become clearly outlined and begins to have a firmer body mass, the vesicle in question becomes fleshier and stronger, changes its disposition and extends to the auricles, above which the body of the heart begins to increase in size, though as yet performing no public duty. When, however, the foetus has been formed, and the bones have now become distinct from the fleshy parts, and the animal has been completed and can be felt to have movement, then it has also within it a pulsating heart which, as I have said, transfer the blood by means of both ventricles from the vena cava into the aorta.

Thus Nature, perfect and divine, making nothing in vain, has neither added a heart unnecessarily to any animal nor created a heart before it had a function to fulfil, but by the same steps in the formation of every animal, that is to say, by going through the patterns available in all animals (egg, worm, foetus) she secures perfection in the individuals. In respect of the formation of the foetus, the points mentioned here are to be confirmed elsewhere by a series of observations.

Finally, it was not without justice that Hippocrates in his book,

De Corde, styled the heart a muscle, for it has an identical action and office, namely, to contract and to move something, in this case the blood contained within it. Further, as in the muscles proper, one can envisage the action and office of the heart from the arrangement of the fibres and the underlying structural basis of movement. According to all the anatomists from Galen up to the present time, the body of the heart is composed of variously coursing fibres, namely, straight, transverse and oblique, but in fact in a boiled heart the arrangement of fibres is found to be other than this. All the fibres in the walls and the septum are circular as in a sphincter, but those in the 'armlets' of muscle have their long axes set at an angle to the long axes of the circular fibres. Hence, when all the fibres contract simultaneously, the apex is drawn towards the base by the 'armlets', the walls come together concentrically, the heart contracts down everywhere, and the ventricles are narrowed. So, as the heart's action is a contraction, its function must be regarded as being the extrusion of the blood into the arteries.

We must equally agree with Aristotle's view about the pre-eminence of the heart, and refrain from asking if it receives movement and sensation from the brain and blood from the liver, if it is the source of the veins and of the blood and so forth. For those who attempt to refute Aristotle with such questions disregard or do not appreciate the chief point, namely, that the heart is the first part to exist and that it was the seat of blood, life, sensation and movement before either the brain or the liver had been created, or had appeared clearly, or at least had been able to perform any function. With its special organs designed for movement the heart, like some inner animal, was in place earlier. Then, with the heart created first, Nature wished the animal as a whole to be created, nourished, preserved and perfected by that organ, to be in effect its work and its dwelling-place. Just as the king has the first and highest authority in the state, so the heart governs the whole body. It is, one might say, the source and root from which in the animal all power derives, and on which all power depends.

But there are also very many points about the arteries which similarly illustrate and bear out the truth of my contention. For instance, Why does the vein-like artery not pulsate, though it is numbered among the arteries? or, Why is a pulsation felt in the artery-like vein? The answer to both questions is that the inthrust of blood into the arteries is the cause of their pulsation[, and such inthrust occurs into the latter vessel, but not into the former one]. Again, one is asked, Why do the arteries differ so much from the veins in the thickness and strength of their walls? To this the reply is that it is the arteries which bear the brunt of the heart's vigorous outthrust and of the blood's violent inflow. Hence, as perfect Nature makes nothing in vain and is sufficient in all respects, the nearer the arteries are to the heart the more they differ in structure from the veins, and the stronger and more ligamentous they are than these. On the other hand, in their most distant disseminations, such as those in the hand, foot, brain, mesentery, and the spermatic ones, the two sets of vessels are so similar in structure that it is difficult, from a visual inspection of their coats, to distinguish one from the other. This is, however, justly so, for the farther the arteries are from the heart, the much smaller is the force with which they are struck by the cardiac impulse, weakened as it is by the great distance which it has travelled. Further, though the impulse in question must have been adequate for the blood in all the arterial trunks and their branches, it is reduced by some fraction at each division so that the ultimate hairlike arterial branches seem to be veins not only in structure but also in function. For their perceptible pulsation is either nil or intermittent, and even in the latter case occurs only when the heart beats with unusual violence, or an arteriole is dilated or overwidely open in some small section. It is on this account that we are able, at some times but not at all times, to feel a pulsation in the teeth and in swellings, and in the fingers. Children always have quick and rapid pulses, hence it is only through the sign which I have mentioned that I have seen for certain that they were labouring under fever. Similarly in tender and delicate subjects I have readily been able, by pressing on the fingers, to ascertain from the digital pulse the time of a febrile attack. On the other hand, when the heart beats over-languidly, it is not only in the fingers but also in the wrist or temples that I have failed to detect a pulse; this I have experienced in cases of fainting, of onset of hysterical symptoms, and of asphyxia, also in over-weak subjects and in those about to die.

At this point, to prevent them from being misled, surgeons should be reminded that in amputation of limbs, excision of fleshy swellings, and treatment of wounds, blood escaping with force is always coming from an artery, but it does not always escape in jets since the small arteries are devoid of pulsation, particularly if they have been compressed by a ligature.

Further, one and the same reason supplies the answer to the double question, Why does the artery-like vein not only have the structure and coat of an artery, but also differ so much less from the veins, in respect of the thickness of that coat, than the aorta does? The reason is that the aorta sustains a stronger inthrust of blood from the left ventricle than the artery-like vein does from the right ventricle. The latter's coats are also softer in texture than those of the aorta to the same extent that the right ventricle of the heart is weaker-walled and less fleshy than the left one. There is, in addition, as much difference between the coat of the artery-like vein and that of the aorta as there is, in respect of texture and of softness, between the lungs and the general system of the body, muscles included. Throughout all the different features, therefore, the same proportionate standard is retained. As human subjects rise in the scale of brawniness, muscularity, and toughness of build, and their hearts in that of strength, thickness, compactness and provision of fibres, so do their auricles and arteries exhibit a corresponding, proportionate increase in thickness and strength and all other respects. On the other hand, animals in which the ventricles of the heart are internally smooth, devoid of villi and valves, and thinner-walled (for example, fishes, birds, serpents, and very many kinds of other animals), all possess arteries which differ little or not at all from the veins in respect of the thickness of their coats.

Further questions are, Why do the lungs have vessels, vein and artery, of such large size that the trunk of the vein-like artery is greater than the two femoral and jugular branches, put together? and Why are the lungs stuffed so full of blood, as from experience and my own personal observation I know them to be? With Aristotle's warning in mind, I was not misled through looking at lungs that I had removed from experimental animals after they had lost all their blood by haemorrhage. The answer to the questions, in any case, is that the lungs and the heart contain the storehouse, source and treasury of the blood, and the laboratory in which it is brought to perfection. A related question is, Why in making an anatomical dissection do we find the vein-like artery and the left ventricle so very full of blood which is identical with that filling the right ventricle and the artery-like vein and, like it, dark in colour and tending to clot? The reply is that the blood passes through the lungs from the latter site to the former one. Two final queries are, first, Why does the artery-like vein, as it is commonly called, have the structure of an artery and the vein-like artery that of a vein? The answer is that, contrary to general belief, the former is in truth an artery, and the latter a vein, both functionally and structurally and indeed in every respect. The second query is, Why has the artery-like vein so wide an opening? and the answer to it is, Because it carries much more than is necessary for the nutrition of the lungs.

All these phenomena to be seen during dissection, and very many others, appear if rightly assessed to elucidate well and to confirm fully the truth which I stated earlier in this book, and at the same time to oppose the commonly accepted views. For it is very difficult for any one to explain in any other way than I have done the reason why all these things have been arranged and carried into effect in the manner that I have described.

LETTERS AND ESSAYS ON THE CIRCULATION OF THE BLOOD

A LETTER FROM WILLIAM HARVEY TO CASPER HOFMANN

Your frank opinion of me, my learned Hofmann, and of the movement and circulation of the blood, was very pleasant to me, and I rejoice at having seen and spoken with a man so learned, whose affection I so gladly accept as to return it. First you thought fit to indict me rhetorically, and tacitly to censure me because I seemed to you to charge and convict Nature of folly and of error, and to characterize her as a very stupid and idle worker to the extent that she would let the blood recrudesce, and with a view to its concoction let it return again and again to the heart, and with a view to its recrudescence equally often to the body in general, and this with the object that Nature, in order to have something to do, may uselessly destroy the formed and perfected blood. But indeed, as I am quite unaware where or when I said and thought such things, and as I have always been full of admiration for Nature's skill, wisdom, and industry, I was not a little upset to have been given such a reputation by a man so very fair-minded as yourself. In my published booklet I simply assert that there is a continuous and uninterrupted movement of blood from the heart through the arteries to the body as a whole, and likewise back from that body as a whole through the veins to the heart, with such flow and ebb that in such quantity and amount that it must somehow move in a circle. But with respect to the coction and the causes of this movement of circulation, especially with respect to its final cause, you will find it clearly stated (if you will kindly re-read Chapters VIII and IX) that I have made no mention, indeed, that I have deliberately quite forgone any discussion of these matters.

Nay more, you proceed to find fault with me as being too little of an analytical anatomist in that I try to investigate the final cause without establishing the facts, I shall be grateful, my frank and very well-wishing friend, if you will read the summary of the whole of my assertions in Chapter XIV. You will be able to discover that I give merely the facts and add no physiological speculation or extra causes, nor the reason why Nature produces this movement of the blood through the pulsation of the heart. I do not deny that in Chapter VIII I insert incidentally for the sake of illustrating what might well happen that the parts are nourished from the heart through the inflow of heat in the blood, and that contrariwise the blood is impaired or undergoes something in the parts so that to recover again its perfect state it seeks once more the heart and source of its warmth. But I do not claim to have shown whether or not this is so or to have said very much about it. Similarly in the last chapters I concluded from the consequences and from my anatomical observations that a circulation probably occurs though I nowhere give causes for such (save for the movement of the heart and for its pulsatile power).

By way of demonstration, since you crave ocular evidence, the circulation of the blood has been clearly described everywhere, and I now declare to you that I have also seen it clearly with my own eyes, and that I have very often demonstrated it by repeated vivisections to very clear-sighted folk among very many most learned men, that the blood moves from the veins to the ventricles of the heart, and thence through the arteries by means of the heart beat to the body as a whole, and finally from the parts of that whole the blood seeks out the heart by means of the veins, and that in such amount and with so vigorous a flow that there appears to be no place left for doubt about a circulation.

But bear me no ill-will, I pray, that I, as an anatomist (and a thinking animal) make use of reasons derived from sensation and taken from the selected admissions of anatomists as a whole, not for the sake of a rhetorical exercise but to confirm, probably, for those who have never visually examined anatomy or who shun such sights, a statement of fact deriving from an autopsy. Can it displease you that Primrose is making calculations on the same lines as I myself, since anatomists as a whole acknowledge that systole and diastole, or constriction and dilatation, do occur in the heart and in dilatation the blood received from the vena cava fills the dilated heart and in its constriction they cannot deny that blood is transfused into the arteries (as they have been taught by the texture of the organ and the cunning device of the valves and many other things about the heart). If any transmission of blood occurs in any amount in individual pulsations, let them suppose whatever quantity they wish (I am not referring to how much I saw), immediately convinced on this basis by the computed pulsations, they must agree that the blood goes around. If, however, you wish to see and feel for yourself how much the single constrictions of the heart account for, and see with your own eyes facts which can make your belief more certain, what happened to me will be as surely, clearly, and evidently apparent (with the techniques properly carried out) as you know you saw yesterday at Altdorf, and I am as certain that the blood is diffused through the arteries into the body as I am certain that our Thames falls into the sea, and within the smaller veins to the larger ones and to the base of the heart from the body as a whole, with such free passage and confluence as your Pegnitz flows into your Regnitz or your Main and Moselle into the catchment of the Rhine.

Up to this point the opinion of a very good man has spoken against me personally rather than against the circulation. For granted that I am not much of an anatomist, and a very bad analyst, and it appears to an upright and learned man that I have slandered Nature, it does not therefore follow that the circulation of the blood is non-existent. You are wrong, my very dear friend, if you judge me so vainly obstinate on behalf of that or any other opinion that I am quite unable to bear contradictory words (especially from my Hofmann, to the sight of whom I had so looked forward that I could not in any way miss the chance of seeing him, whose friendly discourse used so to delight me, and whose letters, written in his own hand, now bring me so great joy). Indeed, there have not been wanting in England such people as have striven in their public anatomy lectures to deny me the discovery of the blood circulation and (quoting your writings) have taught that I was indebted to your training and instruction for my doctrine so that I had to compare our letters and dates in order to defend and clear myself. Finally, I accept gratefully and favourably your [conclusion] that the blood in its vessels is not like water in its aqueducts or our Thames rolling its streams in their channel straight to the ocean, but (as the great Scaliger more correctly interprets the fluctuation in Aristotle which, you say, holds me captive), as there is always some flow of water in a pond or in the sea, and as the river-bank takes up moisture in no small amount by absorption, so the parts requiring nourishment are ever thirsty. But I shall be happy, my dear and learned friend, if you now take your hammering. Does water flow in ponds? (You will forgive me, but I do not understand.) Or does it flow as in the sea? A suspect alternative, but supposing it does flow as in the sea?

there is a flow and ebb at set times and equally the blood must penetrate and return in its vessels and Nature would wish [something] distinct and definite rather than indefinite and confused in her vessels. Moreover, why do the lands of Egypt not get such moisture from the Nile as it flows past, just as if it were inundating? I do not grasp it. Equally how the nourishment drawn off in the effluent blood adheres and is changed into cambium escapes me. The remainder of the doubts advanced in your letters against a circulation are there because you boggle at porosities and blind meanderings of the flesh. The method of passing and possible routes for which you ask are frankly hindrances to the contrary movements of expulsion and retention and you seek the final cause and you say the solution of doubts [is] a sigh of a perfectly constituted truth. The heart draws from the liver, why is this latter's attractive and retaining power no obstacle to you? And by what ways and vents, by anastomosis, or directly through the parenchyma of the liver can the blood reach the cava from the mesenteric veins? You have never seen it but you have no doubt that it is so. Does the liver raise nutriment from the narrow and capillary branching of the portal vein and at one and the same time is blood distributed quite unimpeded to the intestines? You cannot stop me by affirming a contrariety of movements or a confusion. But I fear lest, if I were to reply to single points, this page would expand into a volume and I should overmuch abuse your patience. And listen, either you did not pay attention to my booklet in reading it or you forgot so to do. But do you not grasp the book? Or unless my memory is at fault your objections raised here have their answers treated of in the book and do not refute me. For the man is not to be rejected who admits the circulation through autopsy or probable proof, even if he does not know the routes or facilities, for such inquiry comes later, and contradiction from such things is too argumentative. But since you seek solutions so that I could free you from your doubts, and not to prevent your allowing the cause itself, I promise them, but more correctly according to analytical science when you know the facts correctly and acknowledge them.

Now I fear lest you truly judge me too little of an analyst, assigning causes or solving doubtful points for him who will not admit the existence of the facts; for it is a sophistical way and like speculating about the non-existent; my fingers are already painfully tired from holding the pen and other matters call me away. I have wanted to say these things in order to remove misunderstanding and to free myself from the disrepute of censure on such a scale, and I beg you, most learned and fair-minded friend, if you wish to see with your eyes anything that I affirm about the circulation, just to let me know the facts and I guarantee, as is more becoming in an anatomist, to be present whenever you wish and I am given the opportunity. If, however, you are unwilling for this, or it does not please you to investigate by your own efforts in dissection, at least, I adjure you, refrain from despising the industry of others or turning it into a fault, and do not refuse to trust an honest man, who is not unskilled or mentally deranged, in respect of something which he has tested so often over so many years.

Now farewell and take care to act as I do, for I am accepting your letter in the frank and friendly spirit in which you say that you wrote it. Do you also treat me similarly as I reply to you with equal good-will. Nuremberg, 20 May 1636.

Your

WILLIAM HARVEY, Physician to the King and Professor of Anatomy at the College of Physicians of London. Englishman.

THE FIRST ANATOMICAL ESSAY TO JEAN RIOLAN ON THE CIRCULATION OF THE BLOOD

Not many months ago there appeared a small anatomical and pathological work written by the distinguished Riolan, and I acknowledge very gratefully the author's personal gift of a copy to myself. I certainly congratulate him on his happy choice of so outstandingly praiseworthy an object for his investigations. To demonstrate the seats of all diseases is a task demanding an altogether unusual capacity, and certainly the man who reveals those diseases which all but defy comprehension has undertaken a difficult task. Such efforts become the leading anatomist, for there is no knowledge except that which is based on pre-existing perception, and no certain and fully accepted idea which has not originated from sensation. For this reason the subject itself, and the example set by so great a man, kept demanding a corresponding activity on my own part, and determining me to indite and commit to writing in similar fashion my medical anatomy also, that is, my anatomy most closely adapted to medical use. This was not solely, as in Riolan's case, for the purpose of showing from the cadavers of healthy subjects the sites of diseases and of listing what others had thought must be the appearances of diseases in those places. But it was rather so that from many dissections of patients dying of very severe and remarkable complaints I should undertake an account of the ways and manners in which the internal parts change in site, size, constitution, figure, substance, and other appreciable variables from the natural form and appearance commonly described by all anatomists, and the various remarkable ways in which they are affected.

For just as the dissection of healthy and well-conditioned bodies is of very great help in advancing natural knowledge and correct physiology, so is the inspection of diseased and cachectic bodies of very great assistance in the understanding of pathology. The contemplation of those things which are normal is physiology, and it is the first thing to be learned by medical men. For that which is normal is right and serves as a criterion for both itself and the abnormal. By defining in its light departures from it and unnatural reactions, pathology becomes more clearly obvious for the future, and from pathology the practice and art of therapeusis, and opportunities for discovering multiple new remedies, derive. Nor would one readily believe the extent to which the inner parts are corrupted in diseases, especially those of long standing, and what horrible monstrosities are produced in those parts by diseases. And, if I may so state, one dissection and opening up of a decayed body, or of one dead from chronic disease or poisoning, is of more value to medicine than the anatomies of ten people who have been hanged.

This does not mean that I disapprove the schema advanced by the very learned and skilful anatomist, Riolan. On the contrary, I regard it as extremely praiseworthy for, in as much as it throws light on the physiological aspect, it is very useful to medicine. I thought, however, it would be no less profitable to the art of healing were I to reveal not only the sites affected but at the same time the affections of those sites, describe what I had seen in them, and put on record my findings derived from my many dissections.

The passages in Riolan's booklet, however, which appeared to refer to me only, namely, the accounts of the blood-circuit discovered by me, are the matters which need first consideration, especially by myself. For Riolan is easily the leader and doyen of all contemporary anatomists, and the judgment of so great a man upon so major a subject cannot be lightly esteemed. Rather is his approval more important than the acclaim of all other critics, his censure more deserving of respect and consideration than the opposition of all others in the field. In Book 3, Chap. 8, then, of his *Encheiridium*, he accepts my movement of the blood in animals, sides with me, and adopts my view about the blood circuit. He does not however, do so fully and openly, for in Book 2, Chap. 21, he says that the blood contained in the portal vein does not circulate in the way that that in the vena cava does. Then in Book 3, Chap. 8, he says that there is a circulation of blood, and the circulatory vessels are presumably the aorta and vena cava. He denies, however, that their branches get a circulation. 'For' he says, 'the blood poured out into all parts of the second and third region remains in them for their nourishment and does not flow back into the larger vessels unless it is compelled thereto by the extreme dearth of blood in those vessels, or flows to them in the excitement of a frenzied rush.' And a little farther on he writes, 'so the blood in the veins is constantly ascending naturally or flowing back to the heart, while the blood in the arteries is descending or passing away from that organ. However, if the smaller veins of the arms and legs are emptied of blood, the blood in the veins can descend as the vessels are successively depleted. This I have clearly demonstrated, contrary to the belief of Harvey and of de Wale.' And, as Galen and daily experience confirm the anastomoses of veins and arteries, and there is need for a circulation of blood, 'you will see', he says, 'how such a circulation takes place without causing upset and mixing of the body's humours and destruction of traditional medicine'.

These words reveal the motives actuating this distinguished scientist so that he wished in part to acknowledge, in part to deny, a circuit of the blood; they show that the reason for his hesitant and variable opinion in the matter is his fear of destroying traditional medicine. It was not love of the truth (which he could not have missed seeing) which led him to refrain from speaking freely, but rather excessive caution lest he should offend traditional medicine, or perhaps appear to retract from the physiology he himself put forward in his *Anthropologia*. For the concept of a circuit of the blood does not destroy, but rather advances, traditional medicine. It goes against the [current] physiology of the physicians and their speculation about natural matters, and contradicts anatomical teaching about the functional anatomy of the heart and lungs and remaining viscera. That these things are so will readily be apparent from Riolan's own words of avowal, in part also from the arguments which I here subjoin. These are that the whole of the blood, wherever it is in the living body, moves and alters its position (whether it is within the larger vessels and their offshoots and divisions, or within the porosities of any region of the body's parts), and flows both to the heart and away from it continuously and uninterruptedly, and stays nowhere without loss, though I grant that in places and from time to time it moves forward relatively more rapidly or more slowly.

In the first place, then, the learned gentleman merely denies, without proving his point, that the blood contained in the offshoots of the portal vein circulates. Nor could he have made such denial had he not minimized the strength of his own evidence [to the contrary]. For in Book 3, Chap. 8, he says that if the heart takes in at each beat one drop of blood and expels it into the aorta, and if within the hour it beats two thousand times, then a large part of the blood must pass [through the organ in question in the time stated]. He must make a similar admission with respect to the mesentery. For at each heartbeat more than one drop of blood is forced in through the coeliac artery and the mesenteric arteries and driven into the mesentery and its veins. It must, therefore, get out again somewhere in like amount, or else the branches of the portal vein must in time be disrupted. And one cannot (to resolve the difficulty) regard as probable or possible an Euripus-like inflow and outflow of the mesenteric blood, through one and the same set of vessels, in useless ineffective activity. Nor is it likely that blood passes through these same vessels to discharge into the aorta, for this it cannot do against the force of the blood entering the vessel in the opposite direction. And alternation in flow is not possible where inflow is so definitely continuous, uninterrupted, and unceasing, but, just as is the case with the heart, so blood driven into the mesentery must get out elsewhither. As is obvious, for Riolan could upset all idea of a circulation by the same specious argument if he makes the like declaration with the same amount of probability in speaking about the ventricles of the heart. Namely, if he says that in the systole of the heart the blood is driven into the aorta and in its diastole flows back [into the ventricles]; and the aorta empties itself into the ventricles of the heart as the ventricles of the heart in their turn into the aorta. And so there is a circulation neither in the heart nor in the mesentery, but there is an alternate flux and reflux in ineffective effort. If, therefore, in the heart for the reason approved by Riolan there is of necessity a circulation of blood, the same force of argument holds good also in respect of the mesentery. If, however, there is no circuit of blood in the mesentery, there is similarly none in the heart. For both declarations, namely, the one about the heart and the other about the mesentery, stand or fall similarly by virtue of the same evidence with merely the words changed.

Riolan says 'the sigmoid valves prevent backflow in the heart, but there are no valves in the mesentery'. To which I reply that this too is untrue, for a valve has been found in the splenic vein and often also in other veins. Moreover, valves are not required everywhere in veins, and they are not found in the deep veins of the limbs but rather in the skin vessels. For what need is there of valves where the blood is flowing naturally down from smaller branches to larger ones, and is adequately or more than adequately prevented from flowing backwards by the pressure of the surrounding muscles, but is forced on to where a way lies open to it? Moreover, the amount of blood driven into the mesentery at each pulsation can be calculated if you compress at the wrist with a medium-tight ligature the veins emerging from the hand and going up amongst the arteries, and remember that the arteries of the mesentery are larger than those of the wrist. If you count the number of pulsations required to distend the vessels of the hand and cause the hand as a whole to swell up, then divide by that number and do a little arithmetic; you will find that at each beat, unhindered by the ligature, more than a drop of blood goes in and is prevented from coming out again. Nay, rather, by filling up in this way [the arteries] the blood forcibly distends the whole of the hand and makes a mass of it. By analogy one can infer that the mesenteric blood inflow is as great or greater in proportion as the mesenteric arteries exceed in size those of the wrist. And, if one looks and thinks how much difficulty and effort are involved, and what compresses, ligatures, and apparatus of all sorts are needed to confine the headlong outrush of blood from a cut or tear in even the smallest arteriole, how forcibly (as if shot out by a pipe) it ejects, expels, or saturates all the means taken to deal with it, he will, I think, scarcely believe it probable that any backflow can take place without opposition of this order against so great an impulse and inflow of blood. Turning all of which over in his mind, therefore, I hardly think he will bring himself to believe that against so violent and powerful an inflow the blood from the branches of the portal vein percolates through the same channels to empty the mesentery.

Moreover, if the learned gentleman thinks that the blood does not move in a circle and change, but stagnates unaltered in the branches of the mesentery, he seems to suppose that there are two different blood supplies serving different functions and purposes, and therefore of different nature, in the portal vein and vena cava. The one needs a circulation for its own preservation, the other does not. This is not apparent, nor does he demonstrate that it is true.

Further (*Encheiridium*, Book 2, Chap. 18), he adds 'a fourth kind of vessels to the mesentery; these are styled lacteals and were discovered by Aselli'. With them added to the picture, he appears to imply that all the food extracted by the intestines is carried by these lacteals to the liver, where the blood is manufactured. In the liver the food is digested and changed into blood (as he says in Book 2, Chap. 8) and 'this blood is carried from the liver and passes across to the right ventricle of the heart. With these vessels accepted', he says (*ibid.* Book 2, Chap. 18), 'all the difficulties, that previously arose about the distribution of chyle and blood through the same channel, cease. For the lacteal vessels carry the chyle to the liver and' are channels in their own right, and 'can be separately obstructed'. But how indeed, I ask, can that milk be transfused and cross over into the liver, and thence through the cava into the ventricle of the heart (since the learned gentleman denies that the blood contained in the very numerous branches distributed to the snub-nosed porta hepatis can cross to bring about a circulation)? May I be told how this can be shown possible, especially since blood appears more spirituous and penetrative than the chyle or milk contained in those lacteal vessels; and is so driven on by the pulsation of the arteries that it finds a way elsewhither?

The learned gentleman makes mention of a certain treatise of his about the circulation of the blood. I would that I could see it. Perhaps I would change my mind. But if the learned gentleman had preferred, I do not see but that, having granted the circular movement of the blood (in the veins, as he says in Book 3, Chap. 8, the blood goes continuously and naturally up to the heart or flows down to the heart; just as in all the arteries the blood descends or leaves the heart), with this movement – I say – granted, all the difficulties which used to arise about the distribution of the chyle and the blood through the same channels, would equally cease to exist, so that there would be no further need to search for or suppose separate vessels for the chyle. Seeing that, just as the umbilical veins absorb the nutrient juice from the fluids of the egg, and carry it off for the nourishment and increase of the chick, now existing as the embryo, so do the mesenteric veins drive the chyle from the intestines and carry it to the liver; and why do we hesitate to postulate the same function in the adult? For all the difficulties that used to arise vanish if we assume not two opposing movements, but one continuous one in the mesenteric vessels from the intestines to the liver.

I shall state elsewhere what I must feel about the lacteal veins when I deal with the milk which I have recently found in various parts of newborn animals, especially human ones. For it is found in the mesentery and all its glands, also in the thymus, and in the axillae and the breasts of infants. This milk the midwives get rid of, as they think, for the good of the offspring.

Moreover, the learned Riolan has not only decided that the blood in the mesentery lacks a circulation, but he also asserts that the same is true of the branches of the vena cava and of the arteries and of all the parts of the second and third region, so that the only circulatory vessels which he names are the vena cava and the aorta. In Book 3, Chap. 8, he gives a very weak reason, namely, 'that the blood poured out into all parts of the second and third region remains in them for their nutrition, and does not flow back into larger vessels except it is removed by force and through extreme dearth of blood in the larger vessels, or through a sudden rush flows into the circulatory vessels'.

It is indeed necessary that the portion which is to go off for nutrition should remain. For it would not nourish were it not assimilated in place of that which has been lost, and did it become adherent to the rest and fuse with it. But it is not necessary for the whole of the inflowing blood to remain there for the conversion of only so small a portion of it. For no part uses for its food as much as it contains all told in its arteries, veins, and porosities. It is also unnecessary for it to leave any nutriment behind during its flux and reflux, so in order to nourish it does not all have to remain behind. But the learned gentleman, in the very booklet in which he states this, appears almost everywhere to declare strongly the opposite, especially where he is describing the circulation in the brain and says 'in so far as the brain sends blood back through the circulation to the heart and so the heart is cooled'. In this way all the distant parts may be said to cool the heart. Whence also in fevers when the praecordia are violently consumed and burn with febrile heat, the patients remove their clothing and discard their bedding in their search for cooling for the heart. While, as the learned gentleman states in respect of the brain, the cooled and heat-tempered blood then seeks out the heart through the veins and cools it. In this way the learned gentleman seems to make it more or less obligatory for there to be a circulation from all parts as there is from the brain, a circulation which he had previously openly opposed. But he cautiously and ambiguously asserts that the blood does not return from the parts of the second and third region unless, as he says, it is removed by force and through extreme dearth in the larger vessels, or through a sudden rush flows into the larger circulatory vessels. Which is very true if these words are understood in their true sense. For by the larger vessels in which dearth causes a backflow, I think he must understand the vena cava or the circulating veins, not the arteries. For the arteries are never emptied except into veins or porosities of the parts, but are continuously being distended by the pulsation of the heart. In the vena cava and the circulatory vessels, however, into which the blood slips quickly and hastens to the heart, there would be immediate very great dearth of blood unless all parts incessantly returned the blood poured into them. Add to this that, by the force of the blood which is stretched and driven at each pulsation into all parts of the second and third region, the contained blood is forced from the porosities into the venules and from the branches into the larger vessels, and, moreover, by the movement and pressure of the surrounding parts, for from every container that is compressed and contracted the content is squeezed out. Thus by the movements of muscles and joints the pressure and constraint exerted upon the intervening venous branches push the blood from the smaller into larger vessels.

That the blood, moreover, is continuously and unceasingly driven from the arteries into the individual parts, producing an impulse without backflow, cannot be doubted. If it be admitted that at each pulsation all the arteries are simultaneously distended by the forward drive of blood, and that (as the learned gentleman himself confesses) the diastole of the arteries is produced by the systole of the heart, and that the blood, once it has emerged, never gets back into the ventricles of the heart on account of the closure of the valves; if, I say, the learned gentleman (as it appears) accepts all this, the propulsive force with which the expelled blood is emitted in the individual parts of each region will be obvious. For the inflow and drive reaches everywhere as far as the arterial pulsation extends, whence it is felt in all parts of each region. For pulsation is present everywhere, even in the tips of the fingers and under the nails, and there is no small part at all in the whole body which, suffering from an inflammation or a furuncle, does not feel keenly the lacerating movement of the arterial pulsation attempting to sunder it.

But further, that the blood goes back in the porosities of the parts is obvious in the skin of the hands and feet. For often in severe frost and cold weather we see the hands and limbs so chilled, especially in children, that to the touch they almost give the coldness of ice, and they are so benumbed and stiff as to be almost without feeling and scarcely able to move: meantime, however, they are seen to be full of blood, red or livid. These parts can in no way get warm again except through the circulation, the cold blood deprived of spirits and warmth being driven off and in its place a new, warming, and spirituous blood flowing in from the arteries revives the parts, rewarms them, and restores their movement and sensation. For they could not be refreshed and restored by fire or external heat any more than dead limbs could unless they were revived by the inflow of internal heat. And, indeed, that is the chief use and object of the circulation, and for its sake the blood goes round on its continuous course and perpetual inflow and moves in a circle; namely, so that all parts, depending on it, may be kept by their prime innate heat in life and their vital and vegetative existence, and perform all their functions; while (as physiologists say) they are sustained and actuated by the inflow of warmth and of the spirits of life. Thus, by the help of two extremes, namely, cold and warmth, the temperature of animal bodies is kept in its medium state. For as the inspired air tempers the excessive heat in the lungs and the centre of the body, and looks after the expulsion of suffocating fumes, so in turn does the hot blood, sent through the arteries to the whole of the body, warm all the farthest parts, sustain them and keep them alive, and prevent them from being killed by the power of the external cold.

It would thus be unfair and surprising if individual parts of any region failed to benefit by the transmutation of the blood and the help of the circulation, as Nature appears particularly to have intended by its institution. May I thus conclude? You see how circulation of the blood avoids confusion and disturbance of the humours, both in the body as a whole and in its individual small parts, and both in the larger and in the smaller vessels, and all as is necessary and for the benefit of all parts; without which cooled and weakened parts would never be restored, or remain among the living. For it is clear enough that the protective warmth flows in through the arteries and that its provision constitutes the work of the circulation.

The learned Riolan therefore seems to me to speak more suavely than truthfully when he says in his *Encheiridium* that some parts are without a circulation (doubtless this is with a view to pleasing as many as possible and opposing none) and he seems also to have written with courtesy rather than seriously and with love for the truth. As also he seems to do when he prefers (Book 3,

Chap. 8) the blood to reach the left ventricle through the septum of the heart and certain unknown and vague passages rather than through the very wide and open vessels of the lungs, cunningly furnished with valves preventing backflow. He says he has advanced elsewhere reason for the impossibility and inconvenience of this; I am desirous of seeing it. It would be surprising if the aorta and artery-like vein have the same size, arrangement, and make-up, and not the same function. But it is intensely improbable that the mighty stream of the whole blood-mass should seek out the left ventricle in such force through such small, blind windings through the septum, when the mass in question corresponds to an entry from the vena cava into the right side of the heart and an exit from the left side, both of which need such wide orifices. But our friend has adduced these things inconsistently, for he constitutes the lungs a sort of cleansing channel or outlet for the heart (Book 3, Chap. 6), and says, 'The lung is affected by that blood as it passes through, the sordes of the lung mixing with the blood'. For he says that the 'lungs are corrupted by distempered and ill-conditioned viscera which supply the heart with impure blood, the imperfection of which the heart is unable to emend except through many circuits'. In the same place he says, in opposition to Galen, about blood-letting in peripneumonia and the communication of the veins with the vessels of the lungs: 'If it is true that the blood passes naturally from the right ventricle of the heart to the lungs, to be carried thence to the left ventricle and on again to the aorta; and if the circulation of the blood is admitted; all must see in lung affections that the blood collects in these organs in unduly great amount and overburdens them, unless it is first purged liberally and then in successive portions for the relief of those viscera. This is as advised by Hippocrates, who in swelling of the lung draws blood off from all parts of the body – head, nose, tongue, arms, and feet – so that the amount is reduced and removed from the lung and he draws off blood until the body is bloodless. If a circulation is postulated', he says in the place mentioned, 'the lungs are fairly easily depleted by venesection. If it is rejected, I do not see how the blood can be removed from them. For, if it tries to flow back through the artery-like vein into the right ventricle, the sigmoid valves oppose the movement, while regression from the right ventricle into the vena cava is opposed by the tricuspid valves. So the blood is drawn off through the circulation by section of the arm and leg veins. At the same time,

Fernel's view is upset, namely, that in lung affections it is better to withdraw blood from the right arm than from the left one, because the blood cannot get back into the vena cava except by the rupture of two barriers and of hindrances placed in the heart.'

He adds further in the same place (Book 3, Chap. 6), 'If a ciruclation of the blood be admitted and if it passes usually through the lungs, and not through the median septum of the heart, then the blood circulation must be thought of as twofold. One part is accomplished by the heart and lungs, and in this the blood leaps forward from the right ventricle of the heart and is carried through the lungs to reach the left ventricle of the heart, that is, it has a short course out from a particular viscus and back again into it. The second part of the twofold circulation is through a longer route, beginning with the left ventricle of the heart, passing through the arteries of the whole of the body, and returning through the veins to the right ventricle of the heart.'

It was possible for the learned gentleman here to add a third, very short circulation, namely, from the left ventricle of the heart to the right one, driving a portion of the blood round through the coronary arteries and veins, which are distributed with their small branches through the body, walls, and septum of the heart.

'The person,' he says, 'who admits the one circulation cannot repudiate the other one.' He could equally have added that he cannot deny the third. For to what end should the coronary arteries pulsate in the heart save to drive the blood on by that impulse? And why should there be coronary veins (the office and end of veins being to receive blood brought by arteries) except to acquire the blood from the heart? Add further, that a valve is very commonly found in the opening of the coronary vein [sinus] (as the learned gentleman admits in Book 3, Chap. 9) preventing entry into it, but favouring egress from it. So a third circulation must certainly be admitted by one who admits a general circulation passing through both lungs and brain (Book 4, Chap. 2). Nor, indeed, does he deny that with each pulsation there is an inflow of blood into the individual parts of each region, and an outflow through the veins. And he cannot deny that all small parts are equally recipients of a circulation.

Thus from his very own words it is clear what is the learned gentleman's view both about a circulation of blood through the body as a whole, and about one through the lungs and all other parts. For he who admits the first obviously cannot repudiate the rest. For how can it come about that one who has so often affirmed a circulation through the whole body and through the larger circulatory vessels should deny an universal circulation to any branches, or to any parts of the second or third region? As if all the veins and what he calls the major circulatory vessels were not reckoned by all anatomists, himself included, to be in the second region of the body. Is it possible for there to be a circulation through the body as a whole which does not go through all parts of it? Where he denies it, he therefore acts hesitantly and vacillatingly, giving us empty words. Where, on the other hand, he asserts it strongly, he speaks with judgment and with the addition of solid reasons, as becomes a philosopher. And over and above this view, like a physician of experience and an upright man, he advises – contrary to Galen and his own beloved Fernel – that in very dangerous diseases of the lungs blood-letting is the final remedy. In case of any doubt, I trust that so learned a Christian gentleman may hesitate to recommend to posterity experiments involving the risk of death and decisions about human lives, or to depart without obvious reason from the tenets of Galen and of Fernel, whose opinion he respects most highly. Whatever, therefore, he denies in the blood circuit, whether in the mesentery or in other parts (whether for the sake of the lacteal veins or of traditional medicine or in respect of some other matter), must be attributed to his politeness and modesty and be excused.

Thus far it is, I think, sufficiently clearly apparent, from the distinguished gentleman's words and evidence, that there is a circulation everywhere and that the blood, wherever it is, changes its position and seeks out the heart through the veins. As the learned gentleman shares my views about this, there is no need – indeed, it would be a work of supererogation – to transfer hither my reasons, which I published in my small book on the movements of the blood, for the fuller confirmation of this truth; these reasons deriving from the structure of the vessels, the position of the valves, and other experiments and observations. Especially is this so since I still have not seen the learned gentleman's treatise on the circulation of the blood, nor do I find as yet any proof beyond a bare denial, incited by which he would repudiate in most parts, regions, and vessels a circulation which he admits as universal.

What he discovers as if in justification, from the authority of Galen and daily experience, about the anastomosis of vessels is true. But so great a man (an expert, careful, and diligent anatomist) should first have displayed and shown anastomoses from the larger arteries to the larger veins, these same constituting open and visible gorges proportionate to so great and impetuous a flow of blood mass, and greater than the openings of branches to which he denies a circulation. He was also to be expected to show and declare where they are and how they are constructed, whether they are suitable only for the intromission of blood into veins (as we see the insertion of the ureters into the urinary bladder) and not for reverse flow, or what other wise they were. But (I speak perhaps over-boldly) neither the learned gentleman, nor Galen himself, nor any experience, have ever seen perceptible anasto-moses or been able to demonstrate them.

I myself, with what diligence has been mine to command, have sought hard and have expended not a little of both time and effort in anastomosis exploring. But I have never succeeded in finding vessels, namely, arteries with veins, mutually connecting by inosculation. I would gladly learn from others who ascribe so much to Galen that they swear to his words. [For] there is [in fact] no anastomosis at all in the liver or spleen or lungs or kidneys or any other viscus. When these had been boiled until the whole of the parenchyma had been rendered friable and a sort of powder had been prepared and needled out from all the vascular fibres, I should have been able to see all the fibres of any division and all the capillary threads, had such existed. I dare, therefore, boldly assert that there is no anastomosis of the portal veins with the cava, or of arteries with veins, or of the small capillary branchlets of the bile duct, which are dispersed through the whole moulding of the liver, with the veins. This can be seen in a fresh liver only; all the branches of the vena cava, creeping through the gibbous portion of the liver, have coats riddled with innumerable small holes, as if in a sink constructed for the reception of the blood in its descent. The branches of the portal vein are not similarly arranged, but are divided into offshoots; and both distributions of these vessels, one in the flat part, the other in the gibbous, run everywhere without anastomosis to the portal fissure of the viscus.

In three places, so far as this matter is concerned, I find what is equivalent to an anastomosis. In the brain, from the sleep-producing arteries as they creep through at the basis cerebri, arise numerous interlacing fibres which later form the choroid plexus, and crossing the ventricles end finally by uniting to form the straight sinus which acts as a vein. In the spermatic vessels, commonly called preparative, arterioles originating from the aorta adhere to the so-called preparative veins which they accompany; and at length are taken inside the coats of the veins as if having identical endings, so that where they terminate by the upper part of the testis, the so-called processus coniformis, and corpora varicosum and pampiniforme, it is quite uncertain whether we are assessing the terminations of vein or of artery or of both. In the same way the terminal threads of the arteries going to the umbilical vein are lost in the coats of that vessel.

It cannot be doubted that by such abysses the great arteries, distended and stuffed by the thrust of the blood, would be depleted by so great and conspicuous a torrent. At all events Nature would not have denied perceptible and visible transits, whirls and gorges had she wished to divert thither the whole flow of blood, and hence to prevent the smaller branches and solid parts from profiting by the inflow.

Finally, I will mention this single experiment, which would appear adequate for the demonstration of anastomoses and of their uses (if any) and for upsetting the idea of a [direct] passage of the blood from veins into arteries (through backflow or in other ways).

Open an animal's chest and ligate the vena cava near the heart so that nothing can go into that viscus by that route. Forthwith let the neck arteries be opened up without damage to the veins on either side. If as a result you see the arteries, with their free egress, empty but not the veins, I think it will be obvious that the only route for the blood to be drawn off from veins into arteries is through the ventricles of the heart. For otherwise we should see the veins, like the arteries, emptied of blood in an extremely short space of time (as Galen noted) through the outflow from the arteries.

For the rest, Riolan, I congratulate both myself and yourself, myself because of the significance with which you have invested the circulation, yourself on a learned, polished, and concise book of unsurpassed elegance, for your gift of which to me I thank you most fully, the deserved praises of which I both should and would like to recount; I confess, however, that I am unequal to so great a task. For I know that the name of Riolan inscribed upon the book will carry more honour than the greatest tributes which I may wish. May this little book live in fame for ever and tell the glory of your name to posterity long after even marble has perished. You have most gracefully joined anatomy to pathology and have succeeded in enriching it with a new and very useful osteology. Prosper exceedingly, most distinguished Riolan, and cherish him who wishes you both a long life and a successful one, and hopes that all your very distinguished writings may redound to your everlasting praise,

WILLIAM HARVEY

A SECOND ESSAY TO JEAN RIOLAN

In which many objections to the circuit of the blood are refuted

It is now many years ago, learned Riolan, since with the assistance of the press I published a part of my work. Since that birthday of the circuit of the blood there has of a truth been scarcely a day, or even the smallest interval of time passing, in which I have not heard both good and ill report of the circulation which I discovered. Some tear the as yet tender infant to bits with their wranglings, as undeserving of birth: others by contrast consider that the offspring ought to be nurtured, and cherish it and protect it by their writings. The former oppose it with strong dislike, the latter defend it vociferously. These think that by means of experiments, observations, and my own visual experience I have established the circuit of the blood against the whole strength and force of arguments; the others that it is scarcely as yet sufficiently elucidated, and not yet freed from objections. There are, moreover, those who cry out that I have striven after the empty glory of vivisections, and they disparage and ridicule with childish levity the frogs, snakes, flies, and other lower animals which I have brought on to my stage. Nor do they abstain from scurrilous language.

To return scurrility with scurrility, however, I judge unworthy in a philosopher and searcher after truth. I think it will be better and wiser to tone down these many indications of bad manners by the light of true and trustworthy indications. It is unavoidable that dogs bark and vomit their surfeit, or cynics are numbered among the assembled philosophers, but one must take care that they do not bite, or kill with their savage madness, or gnaw with a canine tooth the very bones and foundations of truth. While I resolved with myself that censurers, mummers, and stain-defiled writers of disapprobations should never be read (as being men from whom nothing sound or remarkable except scurrility was to be expected), I judged them even less worthy of answer. Let them enjoy their evil nature: I think they will scarcely ever have well-disposed readers: and the most good God does not give to the wicked that which is most outstanding and most to be desired, namely, wisdom. Let them continue with their scurrility until it irks if it does not shame them, and finally tires them out.

If with a view to looking at lower animals you wish, if I may so say, to enter the bakehouse with Heraclitus, as told in Aristotle, then do you approach, for the immortal gods are present even here. And the most great Father is sometimes all-powerful in the smallest animals, and more striking in the lower ones. In my book on the movement of the heart and blood in animals I merely brought forward, from many other observations of mine, those by which either errors would be refuted or truth, as I thought, would be best established. Very many other things, to be perceived by the aid of dissection, I omitted as redundant and useless. I will now briefly add some of these for the sake of the studious who earnestly request them.

The great authority of Galen is so all-powerful that I see several hesitate over his experiment about the tying of an artery above a reed introduced into its cavity. The object of the experiment is to show that the pulsation of arteries is brought about by a property transmitted from the heart through their coats, and not by the impact of the blood within their cavities; that, in consequence, arteries increase in volume like bellows and not like bags. This experiment is mentioned by Vesalius, a man very skilled in anatomy, but neither Vesalius nor Galen says that it has been tried by them, as it has by myself. Vesalius just prescribes it, and Galen just advises it, for the information of zealous searchers after the truth, though neither reflects upon or appreciates the difficulties of the task under discussion, or its pointlessness if carried out. For, even if it is done with all due care, it does nothing to confirm the view which asserts that the arterial coats are the cause of the pulsation, but states rather that the exciting cause is the impact of the blood. For, so soon as you have tied the artery above the reed or tube with a string, the vessel in question promptly dilates heartwards from the end of the reed under the impact of the blood from above. In consequence the [forward] flow of blood is impeded and its impact is reflected backwards; the artery subjected to the string-tying pulsates very indistinctly because it lacks the impact of the passing blood the more the latter is reflected backwards above the ligature. If, however, the artery be cut off below the reed, it will be possible to see the opposite from the leap forward of the blood and its expulsion through the reed. As customarily happens (see the note in my small book on the movement of the blood) in an aneurysm, from erosion of the arterial coats, when the blood is contained within membranes, having a container made not from the dilated coats of the artery, but from an unusual surround of membranes and flesh. You may feel the arteries below this sort of aneurysm beat very feebly across it, while above, and especially in the aneurysm itself, large forceful pulsations are seen, though we can imagine that the pulsation and dilatation are produced there not by the coats of the arteries, nor by a property communicated to the container, but clearly from the impact of the blood.

But in order that the error of Vesalius and the inexperience of others may be more clearly seen (they assert their view that the portion of reed submitted to the tying does not beat after it is tied), I myself who have actually tried the experiment say that the portion submitted will [in fact] pulsate if the experiment is correctly carried out. And when you loosen the string, where they assert that the arteries submitted beat backwards, I say that the part submitted to the loosened string beats less than the part submitted to the tied one. But the effusion of blood leaping forward from the wound confuses everything and renders the experiment fruitless and vain, so that nothing definite is demonstrable on account of the impact of the blood, as I have said. But if (as I know from experience) you bare the artery and hold by pressure with the fingers the part you cut, you will be able at will to try many things so that the truth is clear and obvious to you. In the first place, you may at each beat feel the charge of blood coming down into the artery and see it dilating the same. You will also be able, if you relax a small portion of the opening, to express and let go the blood as you wish. It will be obvious to you as you watch closely that the blood shoots out in leaps and bounds at the individual pulsations and (as we said in the account of arteriotomy or of perforation of the heart) is ejected at each contraction of the heart with arterial dilatation. If you allow it to escape in a full continuous flow and permit it to break forth (either through the channel proper or by an opening made in it), you may perceive clearly within the stream itself, both by sight and – if you apply your hand – by touch, all the beats of the heart, and its whole rhythm, order, vehemence, and intermittence. In just the same way as you could distinguish different and varying jets of water squirted through a siphon into the hollow of your hand, so may you perceive, by seeing and feeling it, the varying, uneven impact of the escaping blood. I have on occasion seen it breaking out from a cut neck artery with such force that on striking against the hand, from four or five feet distant, it broke off, rebounded, and recoiled.

But to clear up the point in doubt and show more clearly that the pulsific force does not diffuse through the arterial coats from the heart, I have a span-long portion of a descending aorta with its two femoral branches. It was removed from the body of a very noble gentleman, and it had been turned into a pipe-like bone through the cavity of which, while the very noble gentleman was alive, the arterial blood going down to the feet stimulated the arteries below by its impact. In that case, however, the artery behaved as if it had been constricted and tied above the small fistulous channel, as in Galen's experiment. So that it could neither dilate at that point nor narrow like bellows, nor distribute a pulsific force from the heart to the arteries below and beneath, nor disperse through the solid structure of the bone a faculty which it had not yet received. Nevertheless, I remember very well that I very often observed, during his lifetime, pulsation occurring in the lower part of the artery in the legs and feet. For I was his constantly attendant physician, and he my very close friend. So in that very noble gentleman the arteries below must have been dilated by the impact of the blood like bags, and not by the expansion of their coats like bellows. For the same impediment and same removal of the pulsific property must occur in an arterial coat completely converted into a reed and bony tubelet as in an arterial coat constricting down over a reed and bony tubelet so that the underlying arteries stop pulsating.

I have also known, in another very noble and very powerful gentleman, of the conversion of the aorta, and of the large artery near the heart, into a round bone. So Galen's experiment, or at least its analogue, discovered by chance and not deliberately sought for, shows clearly enough that the impress of the pulsific property is not hindered by constriction or ligation of the arterial coats with consequent lack of pulsation in the underlying arteries. And, if someone duly performed the experiment prescribed by Galen, it would refute the view that Vesalius had hoped would be confirmed by it. I do not, in consequence, deny all movement to the arterial coats, but I admit that which I attribute to the heart, namely, contraction and systole produced from the coats themselves and a reversion to the natural disposition from the state of distension. But it has to be noted that dilatation and contraction are not produced by the same agents, many causes and means being concerned. As one can see in the movement of all parts, and also in the heart itself. It is distended by the auricle, and contracted by its own effort: similarly, the arteries are dilated by the heart, and collapse of themselves.

You will also be able to carry out another experiment at the same time. If you fill two measures of equal capacity, one with outgushing arterial blood, the other with venous blood drawn from a vein of the same animal, you will be able to perceive at once, and also observe afterwards when both bloods have clotted and grown cold, what are the differences between the two. Thereby you will be going against those who imagine a different kind of blood in the arteries from that which exists in the veins. That is, in the former they envisage it more florid, and in some unknown way bubbling up with abundance of spirits, and blown out like milk or honey boiling up over a fire, and swelling up to occupy more room. For if the blood, driven out of the left ventricle of the heart into the arteries, were sufficiently fermented into a frothy, inflated state for a drop or two of it to fill the whole cavity of the aorta, it would doubtless revert to a quantity of some drops with the subsidence of the fermentation (the reason given by some people for the arteries being found empty in the dead); the same would be seen in the receptacle full of arterial blood. This is what we find happens with cooling both in milk and in honey. But, if the blood in each of the two receptacles clots with almost the same coloration and practically the same consistence, expresses its serum similarly, and fills both measures alike during both warming and cooling, this evidence will, I think, suffice to convince anyone (and to stop some folk from going sleepless over the problem) and prove that the blood looks alike in both the left and the right ventricle (as both sense and reason will tell you), for we should have to declare that the vein-like artery has been proportionately distended by one frothy drop, and hence the blood is the same and similarly effervescent and fermenting in the right as in the left ventricle, seeing the entry of the artery-like vein and the exit of the aorta are equivalent and comparable.

Three things are most likely to lead one to this view of the blood's diversity. The first is that in arteriotomy men see a more florid blood withdrawn. The second is that in the dissection of cadavers they find both the left ventricle of the heart and all the arteries equally empty. The third is that they understand that arterial blood is more spirituous and replete with spirits, and thus think of it as occupying much more room. The causes and reasons why these things appear thus are shown by inspection itself.

First, with respect to the colour. Blood, whenever and wherever emerging through a narrow opening, is as it were strained off, and the thinner and lighter part, which tends to float on top and is more penetrative, is forced out. Thus in venesection the blood, breaking forth in greater amount or strength from a relatively large opening and leaping relatively far, is thicker and has more body and is of a darker colour. On the other hand, if it flows out from a small and narrow opening a drop at a time (as it normally does from a vein after a ligature has been removed), it is more florid for it is, so to speak, being strained off, and only the thinner and more penetrative part gets out. The blood is more florid in this way in bleeding from the nostrils, or when it is withdrawn by means of leeches or through cupping-glasses, or gets out how you will by diapedesis. This is because the thick and hard vascular coats become more difficult to negotiate and insufficiently pliant to give free passage to the outgoing blood. It also happens thus in adipose subjects; when the opening of a vein is pressed on by subcutaneous fat, the blood looks thinner and more florid and quasi-arterial. On the other hand, blood flowing freely from a cut artery, when received into a suitable vessel, will look venous. A much more florid blood is found in the lungs and is expressed from them than is found in arteries.

The concept of the emptiness of the arteries in dead bodies (which is perchance that misled Erasistratus into thinking that arteries only contained aërial spirits) derives from the fact that, when the lungs subside on closure of their passages, they are no longer respiring. So the blood cannot pass freely through them. The heart, however, continues for a space of time to force blood out. In consequence, the left auricle of the heart, and the left ventricle, are relatively contracted, and equally the arteries appear empty and devoid of content, being unfilled by their due succession of blood. If, however, at one and the same time the heart ceases to beat and the lungs to give passage for breathing, as in those suffocating by drowning in cold water or dying from syncope and sudden death, you will find the veins and arteries equally filled.

With regard to the third matter, namely, spirits, there are many and opposing views as to which these are, and what is their state in the body, and their consistence, and whether they are separate and distinct from blood and the solid parts, or mixed with these. So it is not surprising that these spirits, with their nature thus left in doubt, serve as a common subterfuge of ignorance. For smatterers, not knowing what causes to assign to a happening, promptly say that the spirits are responsible and introduce them as general *factota*. And, like bad poets, they call this *deus ex machina* on to their stage to explain their plot and catastrophe.

Fernel and others imagine aërial spirits and invisible substances. He proves that there are psychic spirits (in the way Erasistratus proved that there are spirits in the arteries) because small spaces are found in the brain and these, since a vacuum is not acceptable [to Nature], he concludes must be filled during life by spirits. In general, however, the school of physicians agrees on three kinds of spirits, namely, those of growth permeating through the veins, those of life through the arteries, and those of the psyche through the nerves. Hence the physicians say, after Galen, that sometimes the parts work in sympathy with the brain because an ability is restrained with essence, that is, spirit, at other times irrespective of essence. Further, in addition to these three inflowing kinds of spirits, he seems to assert an equal number of stationary ones. I have, however, never found such in veins, nerves and arteries, or parts of living subjects. Some make the spirits corporeal, others incorporeal, and those who want them corporeal sometimes make the blood, or its thinnest portion, the link with the psyche. Sometimes they conceive of the spirits as contained in the blood (like flame in the aroma of cooking) and sustained by its continuous flow; sometimes of the spirits as distinct from the blood. Those who declare the spirits incorporeal have no ground to stand on, but they also recognize capacities as spirits (such as the digestive, chyle-forming, and procreative spirits) and admit as many spirits as they admit faculties or parts.

But the schoolmen also enumerate spirits of fortitude, prudence, patience, and the virtues as a whole, and the most sacred spirit of wisdom, and all divine gifts. Moreover, they suspect that there are bad and good spirits helping, possessing, leaving, and wandering round. They think that illnesses are caused by an evil spirit upsetting the humours. However, though nothing is more uncertain and doubtful than the traditional teaching about the spirits, the majority of physicians appear to end in agreement with Hippocrates, who favoured a tripartite composition of our body, namely, the containing parts, the contents, and the driving factors. These last are interpreted as spirits. But if for driving factors spirits are to be understood, whatever in living bodies has force and drive would be styled spirit. And not all spirits are airy in substance, power and quality: similarly, they are not all incorporeal.

What, however, is specially relevant to my theme after all other meanings have been omitted from consideration as being tedious, is that the spirits escaping through the veins or arteries are no more separate from the blood than is a flame from its inflammable vapour. But in their different ways blood and spirit, like a generous wine and its bouquet, mean one and the same thing. For, as wine with all its bouquet gone is no longer wine but a flat vinegary fluid, so also is blood without spirit no longer blood but the equivocal gore. As a stone hand or a hand that is dead is no longer a hand, so blood without the spirit of life is no longer blood, but is to be regarded as spoiled immediately it has been deprived of spirit. Thus the spirit, which is specially present in the arteries and arterial blood, is either the product of such blood, like wine's bouquet in wine, and the spirit in brandy; or like a small flame kindled in spirit of wine and keeping itself alive on such a diet. In consequence, the blood, though very heavily imbued with spirits, is not turgid with them, nor do they cause it to rise or become blown out so that it wants and needs more space (which, in the experiment already referred to above, you will be able to determine very accurately by measuring the vessels); but, like wine, it is to be understood as prevailing by its superior strength and its vigour in doing and effecting, in the Hippocratic sense.

So the same blood is present in the arteries as in the veins even if it is admittedly more spirituous and more heavily endowed in the former with vital force. It is not, however, changed into something airier or rendered more vaporous, as if there were no spirits save airy ones and no driving forces save windiness and flatulences. But neither are those psychic spirits and those of growth and life, which reside in the solid parts, namely, the ligaments and tendons (especially if there are so many kinds of them), and are contained within blind meanderings, to be regarded as so many different airy forms or kinds of vapours. I would gladly learn from those who acknowledge corporeal spirits in the bodies of animals but give them an airy, vaporous, or fiery consistency, whether those spirits in the absence of blood can cross and flow back and wander hither and thither like separate bodies. I would know, I say, whether the spirits follow the movement of the blood as if they are parts of that fluid or indissolubly . . . bound to it in such a way that they cannot leave the other parts or cross without the blood also flowing in and back and crossing. For if, like the vapours of water attenuated by heat, the spirits from the blood exist in a constant flow and succession as nourishment for the parts, it necessarily follows that they remain near that nourishment but in continuous evanescence, and hence do not flow in or out or cross or remain on the spot without the blood, as their subject, or their carrier, or their nourishment, [likewise] flowing in or out or crossing or remaining on the spot.

May I next learn from those who teach that spirits are made within the heart, and who compound them, by mixing, from the vapours or exhalations of the blood (excited by the heat of the heart or by shaking) and the inspired air, whether such spirits are not to be reckoned much colder than the blood, since both of their component parts, namely, air and vapour, are much colder than it? For the vapour of boiling water is much more bearable than the water itself, and any flame you like burns less than the carbon of a lamp-wick, and wood-charcoal less than red-hot iron or bronze. Thus it would seem that spirits of this sort owe their heat to the blood rather than that the blood is heated by the spirit; that, further, such spirits are to be regarded as soots and outgoing waste products (like smells) rather than as artisans of Nature, especially since they are so frail and short-lived that they would quickly lose their virtue (if they received such at the outset from their blood). Whence it would probably be expiration of the lungs by which the spirits are blown outwards and the blood is aired and purified, while the object of inspiration would presumably be so that the blood, by crossing between the two ventricles of the heart, should be tempered by the cold of its environment, thus avoiding getting overheated and swelling up and being blown out with a kind of fermentation, like honey and milk on the boil, distending the lung to such an extent that the animal was suffocated. I have fairly often seen such in dangerous asthma, where, indeed, Galen gives the cause when he says it results from obstruction of the small arteries (he meant the venous and arterial vessels). I have myself found not a few saved from very real danger of asthmatic suffocation by the application of cupping glasses and the sudden onpouring on to them of a large amount of cold water. What I have said about the spirits is perhaps enough and more than enough in this place; I must define them, and lay down what and of what sort they are, in a physiological treatise.

I will merely add that there are those who treat of innate heat as if of Nature's common instrument for everything, and teach about an inflow of heat to keep all the parts warm and alive, and admit that it cannot exist without a subject but fail to discover a mobile body corresponding to this rapidity of inflow and outflow (especially in mental afflictions) and to the swift movement of this heat. Such writers introduce spirits as highly subtle, extremely penetrative, and mobile bodies, in the same way as they visualize a wonderful divinity of the operations of Nature arising from her common instrument (namely, the innate heat). In like manner, they make out that those sublime, bright, ethereal, celestial, and divine spirits are the bonds of the soul just as the crowd of the ignorant think of the Gods, and proclaim them, as the natural authors of works of which they do not comprehend the causes. Hence they decide that the heat flows constantly into the individual parts through the inflow of spirit, and that that arrives through the arteries: as if the blood could not have been able to move so quickly or penetrate so deeply or warm so greatly. And they are so carried forward by their faith in this view as to deny that blood is contained in the arteries. And they try upon extremely slight evidence to make out that the arterial blood is of a different kind, or that the arteries are filled with aërial spirits of this kind and not with blood, all this in opposition to the arguments advanced by Galen against Erasistratus from both experience and reason. But it is sufficiently clear from the above experiment, and from sense, that the arterial blood is not so different. Sense can equally make it manifest about the inflow of blood, and about spirit not separated from blood (but apparently of the same body) flowing through the arteries.

One can see, when and as often as the extremities of the hands, feet, or ears stiffen with cold and are restored with a fresh inflow of heat, that they simultaneously become coloured, warm, and full, and that the veins, small and forgotten earlier, come into view and swell up. Hence the parts, on suddenly becoming warm again, are sometimes affected by pain. From which it appears that that which on its inflow brings warmth is the same as that which brings fulness and colour. This, however, can be nothing other than blood, as I earlier demonstrated, and (though it needs a relatively long artery and vein) as anyone can so readily appreciate when he sees the nearer (heartwards) portion [of vein] discharge no blood, but the farther one pour out a copious amount, and that of blood alone, in the way recorded later in my experiment on internal jugular veins. When the artery, on the other hand, is divided, little blood emerges from the farther part of the dissection, but the nearer part, as if from a siphon, ejects pure blood with violent force. This experiment decides the hither or thither direction of the flow in each of the two kinds of vessels; it also decides with what speed, what perceptible movement (not gently and drop by drop), and, moreover, what violence. And, lest anyone by way of evasion claims that spirits are invisible, let the opening of the dissected vessel be lowered into water or oil. For, were anything airy to emerge, it would break out through visible bubbles. Since it is in this way that hornets, wasps, and insects of this kind give off at the last as they are dying small bubbles of air from their tails, organs whence it is not improbable that they breathe while alive. For all animals submerged and suffocated in water, when at last they have dissipated their strength and are sinking, commonly give off small bubbles from their mouth[s] and lungs, as they surrender their lives. It is finally shown in the same experiment that the valves shut so perfectly in the veins that inblown air does not get in, let alone blood. It is shown (I say) by sense, and not sensibly or insensibly or gradually or drop by drop, that the blood does not get away backwards from the heart throught the veins.

And lest anyone should have recourse to the statement that these things are so when Nature is upset and preternaturally disposed, but not, however, when she is left to herself and acts freely, since in an ill and preternatural disposition appearances are not the same as in a natural and healthy one – it must therefore be said and thought that although (with the vein divided) it may seem or be stated as preternatural for so much blood to get out of the far portion because Nature is upset, yet the dissection does not close the near part to prevent anything moving out or being pressed out, whether or not Nature is upset. Others quarrel similarly saying that, although (with the artery cut near the heart) the blood promptly begins bursting forth in such amount at each beat, the intact heart and the intact artery do not therefore exert a driving pulsation. However, it is rather possible that each pulse does drive something, and it cannot drive the container without impelling the something contained. However, to defend themselves and avoid a circulation they are not afraid to affirm and assert that in living subjects of healthy habits the arteries are so full that they cannot admit even grains of blood more; so also as regards the ventricles of the heart. But it is beyond doubt that, whenever and how far soever the arteries and ventricles are conceded to contract, they ought to be able to accept some blood sent them by way of an extra, and that amount more than ten grains. For if the ventricles are so distended (as I saw them once in a vivisection) as not to admit any more blood, the heart ceases to pulsate and, remaining tense and resistant, induces death by suffocation.

About the question whether the blood in its movement is drawn or driven or activated by its own inner nature, I have said enough in my small book on the movement of the heart and blood, as also of the way in which the heart's functional activity is expressed as dilatation and contraction: I wrote at the same time about the diastole of arteries. Hence those who take, as evidence of contradicting, the things written there appear either not to understand or to be unwilling to follow up the matter by inspection.

I do not think that anything in the body can be demonstrated as attracted except food, making up gradually for losses by succession of the parts, like lamp-oil attracted by its flame. Hence the first common organ of all sensible attraction and impulsion is that which has the nature of a sinew or of a fibre or of a muscle, namely, that it is contractile and can shorten (by contracting itself), and for that reason can stretch, contract, or drive forward. But I must publish these things more fully and openly elsewhere in connection with the motor organs of animals.

With regard to those who repudiate the circulation because they see neither its effrcient nor its final cause, I have to date added no reply to their query 'Who benefits?', but it still remains to be demonstrated. First, one ought to admit what should be investigated rather than the reason for such further study. For from the things which occur in the circulation and are set down here, the uses and usefulnesses of it should be investigated. Meanwhile, I will say, 'How many things are accepted in physiology, pathology, and therapy of which we do not know the causes, but of the existence of which no one doubts? For example, putrid fevers, revulsion, purgation of excrements. Thus, there are those who set themselves against the circulation because they are unable to solve medical problems with it admitted; or, in curing diseases and using drugs, they are unable to collect thence the causes of appearances; or they fail to see that the causes given them by their teachers are false; or they deem it dishonourable to desert the views they approved; and they consider it impious to throw doubt upon the traditional discipline of so many centuries and the authority of the old. To all these let my reply be that the facts manifest to the senses wait upon no views, the works of Nature upon no antiquity: for there is nothing older or of greater authority than Nature.

Those who raise as impediments to their acceptance of the circulation the insolubility (as they think) of problems deriving from [certain] clinical observations, and who [also] put forward in opposition [to it] their own erroneous statements (for example, that, with the circulation admitted, venesection does not revulse, since the same amount of blood continues to be driven to the part affected) – those who do these things, I say, must fear the passage through that noble and principal viscus, namely, the heart, of excrements and vicious humours, an outflow and an excretion. And sometimes from the same body and different parts, or indeed from the same opening and simultaneously, an evil and corrupt blood emerges though, if the blood were driven by a continuous impulse, it would be shaken up and mixed in its passage through the heart. (They doubt how these things can come to pass, and very many things of this kind from the school of the physicians seem to oppose their acceptance of the circulation. Nor do they think it satisfactory, as in astronomy, to draw up new systems unless they solve all the phenomena.) I will not make any reply here save that the circulation is not everywhere and always the same, but many things happen in consequence of the faster or slower movement of the blood, the strength or weakness of the heart's propulsion, the amount, condition, or constitution of the blood, the density of the parts, hindrance to blood flow, and similar things. A thicker blood passes with greater difficulty through narrow pathways; and it is filtered more in its passage through the parenchyma of the liver than it is through that of the lungs.

It does not course similarly through the rarer texture of flesh and parenchyma on the one hand and through the compact consistence of the sinewy parts on the other. For the thinner and purer and more spirituous part has a more rapid passage; the thicker and the more earthy, ill-humoured, longer-lasting part is rejected. The nutritive part, and ultimate aliment, whether dew or cambium, is more penetrating as universally applicable (even to the horns themselves, feathers, nails, and hairs on all sides if being nourished everywhere they increase in all dimensions); in addition, the excrements are secreted in some places and are stuck together and add to the weight, or are concocted. And I do not consider that excrements (or vicious humours) once segregated, or milk, or the phlegm, or the sperm, or the ultimate aliment (dew and cambium) must necessarily revolve with the blood, but nutriment must adhere in order that it stick together. About all these matters and about very many others to be settled and declared in the proper places, that is to say, about physiology and the remaining parts of the art of medicine, as also about the consequences and inconveniences or conveniences of the circulation of the blood, it is unfitting to dispute before the nature of that circulation itself has been established and admitted as accepted. The example of astronomy is not to be followed here; in this subject, merely from appearances and the actual fact, the causes and the reason why come up for investigation. But (as one seeking the cause of an eclipse would be placed above the moon to discover that cause by sensation and not by reckoning) with regard to sensible things, that is, the things that come under the senses, it will be impossible to bring forward any surer demonstration to induce belief than the actual sensation and seeing for oneself.

There is another remarkable experiment which I wish to have explored by all students of the truth, so that it may be clearly seen that the arterial pulse also has its origin and clarification from the impulse of the blood. If you take what length you will of the inflated and dried intestines of a dog or wolf or other animal (such a preparation as you find in an apothecary's shop), cut it off and fill it with water, and tie it at both ends to make a sort of sausage, you will be able with a finger-tap to strike one end of it and set it a-tremble, and by applying fingers (in the way that we usually feel the pulse over the wrist artery) at the other end to feel clearly every knock and difference of movement. And in this way (as also in every swollen vein in the living or dead body) anyone will be able to teach students, by demonstration and verbal instruction, all the differences occurring in the amplitude, rate, strength, and rhythm of the pulses. For just as in a long full bladder and an oblong drum every blow to one end is felt simultaneously at the other, so in dropsy of the belly, as also in every case of an abscess filled with liquid matter, we are accustomed to distinguish anasarca from tympanites. If every impulse and vibration, produced on one side, is clearly felt by touch on the other, we decide on tympanites; not, as is wrongly thought, because it gives out a drum-sound and is produced only by flatus (which never happens) but because, as in a drum, every rap, even the lightest, passes across and any vibration at all penetrates. For it denotes that there is a serous, and ichorous, and urine-like substance below and not a sluggish or viscid one as in anasarca, which retains the traces of pressure to which it has been subjected, but does not transmit them.

With the introduction of this experiment there arises a most powerful objection to the circulation of the blood which no one who has written against me has noticed or added to the opposition list. For, since in this experiment we saw that systoles and diastoles of the pulse can occur without fluid getting out, will one not suspect that the same may be brought about by the beat of the heart without the need for a circulation, the blood being driven, in Euripus fashion, thence hither and in turn hence thither? But I have elsewhere provided an adequate solution of this difficulty, and now I also say that it cannot be thus in the arteries of the living. For continuously and uninterruptedly the right auricle fills the right ventricle with blood to which the tricuspid valves deny any backflow, and at the same time the left auricle similarly serves the left ventricle. And each ventricle in systole ejects and pushes out blood which the sigmoid valves do not allow to return. Either, therefore, the blood must somewhere continuously and uninterruptedly move on from the lungs and equally from the body arteries or, finally, stagnating and infarcted somewhere, it must either rupture its containing vessels or choke the heart itself by distending it; as I noted its becoming apparent (in my small book on the movement of the blood) in the vivisection of an eel. To clear this doubtful point I will recall two experiments among many others. One of them I have told before: it shows clearly that the blood in the veins is always running towards the heart in a continuous and great effort and flow.

In the exposed internal jugular vein of a doe (in the presence of many nobles and the most serene King, my Master), divided in two across its length, scarcely more than a few drops of blood came out from the lower portion, rising up from the clavicle. On the other hand, through the other opening of the vein a fairly long way down from the head, a round column of blood came out very copiously in a great rush. You will be able to make the same observation daily during the outflow of blood in phlebotomy. For, if you press on the vein with a finger a little below the opening, the outflow of blood is satisfactorily arrested but, on release of the pressure, it flows out again in abundance as before.

In any visible long vein of the elbow, with the hand held up aloft, and all the blood, so far as you can manage, squeezed outwards and downwards, you will see the vein apparently collapsed (with a pitting left in the skin); but, so soon as you press on it with a finger-tip, you will immediately see the part towards the hand fill up, and become turgid and (with blood arriving from the hand) swollen. Why? Because with the breath held and thence the lungs compressed and much air ingested, the vessels of the chest are simultaneously compressed; as a result of this, blood is driven with much redness into the face and eyes. Why? Because (as Aristotle says in *The Problems*) all actions are performed with greater force and strength when the breath is held than when it is released. So a more copious blood is drawn from a forehead or tongue vein when the neck is compressed and the breath is held.

I have sometimes in a recently strangled human cadaver within two hours from its hanging, opened up the chest and pericardium (before the redness of the face had disappeared) and demonstrated to many witnesses the right auricle of the heart and the lungs, greatly distended and infarcted with blood, but especially the auricle, swelling up so to the size of a man's large fist that you would think it would burst. This large mass on the following day, with the cadaver thoroughly chilled and the blood getting lost in other ways, subsided and vanished. So, from these and other experiments, it is adequately shown that the blood proceeds through the veins as a whole to the base of the heart and, unless passage were given, it would be forced into other paths or oppress the heart itself. On the other hand, if it did not flow out of the arteries but were found regurgitating, it would be clear how oppressive it could be.

I will add another observation. A noble baronet, Sir Robert Darcy, a relative by marriage of my dear friend, Doctor Argent, the celebrated physician, often complained when he was about middle age of an oppressive pain in his chest, especially at night time. So that fearing sometimes a syncope, at other times a choking from a paroxysm, he passed a restless and uneasy life. He tried many remedies in vain and consulted all [available] physicians. At length, with his illness worsening, he became cachectic and dropsical and finally, overcome by a violent paroxysm, he died. I examined this patient's cadaver in the presence of Doctor Argent, the then President of the College of Physicians, and of Doctor Gorge, an outstanding theologian and preacher, who was then pastor of that parish. Because of the hindrance to the passage of the blood from the left ventricle into the arteries, the very wall of that ventricle (which seemed adequately thick and robust) had been torn and opened up by a wide rent, for the hole which discharged the blood was of such size that it easily took one of my fingers.

I knew another, prudent man who, for anger and displeasure over a wrong done by someone stronger than himself and over an affront inflicted, became very inflamed and excited. With his ill will and hatred mounting daily because revenge was forbidden, and disclosing to no one the severe mental suffering which so very greatly exasperated him, he at last fell upon a strange kind of disease, and was miserably tormented with very great oppression and with pain in the heart and chest. So that, getting no benefits from the exhibition of the remedies of the most expert physicians, on falling at length after some years into a scorbutic cachexia, he wasted away and died. The only way in which he had been able to get relief had been for the whole of his chest region to be subjected to pressure by a very strong man, and to be kneaded and buffeted as a miller moulds bread (the relief was as frequent and as long-lasting as such treatment). His friends thought him affected by a magician's poison, or obsessed by an evil spirit. This subject's neck arteries, distended to the size of a thumb as though they were respectively the aorta itself or its descending limb, pulsated deeply and strongly and looked like two rather long aneurysms: in view of which I even tried arteriotomy near the temples, but without relief. In the dissected cadaver I found the heart and aorta so distended and stuffed with blood that the cardiac mass and the ventricular cavities stood comparison with, and were equivalent to, the bovine heart in their size. So great is the power of confined or enclosed blood, so dynamic is it.

Although, therefore (as shown in the experiment previously mentioned), an impulse will be able to occur without the fluid finding exit (the water vibrating through the intervening stretch) in the [experimental] sausage to which I earlier referred, the same cannot happen in the vessels of the living without extreme and very serious hindrances and dangers. However, it is clear from the facts set down that the blood does not pass everywhere with the same speed and rapidity, and equally not with the same vehemence, in all places and parts and at all times. But it varies greatly according to age, sex, temperament, habit of body, and other contingent internal or external, and natural or unnatural, circumstances. For it does not pass with the same rapidity through occluded, obstructed, or impeded paths and meanderings as it does through open, free, and patent ones, nor through bodies or parts that are dense, constricted, and infarcted as it does through those that are thinner, relaxed, and free from obstructions. Nor, when the impulse occurs weakly, slowly, and gently does it run forward or penetrate so quickly as it does when it impinges with force and strength, and is driven with vehemence and in quantity. Nor is the blood itself when it is thickened or made more solid or more earthy, so penetrative as it is when it is more serous, thin, and more liquid. Hence it is more reasonably supposed that the blood in its circuit crosses more slowly through the kidneys than through the substance of the heart; more rapidly through the liver than through the kidneys; through the spleen than through the liver; through the lungs than through the muscles or through any other viscera according to the comparative rareness of their compositions.

We can similarly think about age, sex, temperament, and habit of body, soft or hard; about the body-condensing action of the cold of the surrounding air, when the veins are scarcely visible in the limbs, or a red colour perceived or heat felt; and about the blood, made more liquid by the accession of aliment from the food. Thus, too, veins are noticeably more liberal with their blood in venesection from a warm body than they are from a cold one. We see how, if a frightened patient faints from mental anxiety during a venesection, the outflow of blood stops at once and a bloodless pallor overspreads the whole surface of the body, the limbs become rigid, there is whistling in the ears, and the eyes are afflicted by blindness. I find a field in which I can roam over-far and digress too widely. For so great a light of truth shines out for the explanation of so many problems, for the solution of so many doubts, for the investigation of the causes of so many affections and diseases and therapeutic opportunities that they would appear to demand a special treatise. From all these I shall deal in my medical observations with those worthy of remark.

For what is more remarkable than the way in which our body reacts differently in every affection, appetite, hope, or fear, and the countenance itself changes, and the blood appears to be escaping hither or thither? The eyes redden with anger and the pupil is constricted. In bashfulness, the cheeks are lavish with blushes; in fear, disgrace, and shame, the face is pale but the ears are red as if about to hear ill: in adolescents touched with desire, how quickly is the penis filled with blood, erected and extended? But what is most worthy of observation by physicians and most useful, why do blood-letting and the exhibition of cupping glasses, and compression and artificial construction of the artery taking the blood flow to a part (especially while the change is actually being made) assuage and remove all pain as by a charm? These matters, I say, must be referred to my *Observations*, where they are unravelled and clarified.

Silly and inexperienced persons wrongly attempt, by means of dialectics and far-fetched proofs, either to upset or to establish which things should be confirmed by anatomical dissection and credited through actual inspection. Whoever wishes to know what is in question (whether it is perceptible and visible, or not) must either see for himself or be credited with belief in the experts, and he will be unable to learn or be taught with greater certainty by any other means. Who will persuade those who have never tasted it that wine is sweet and far surpasses a drink of water? With what proofs will he convince those who are blind from birth that the sun is bright and more splendid than all the stars? So [also] about the circuit of the blood, which all have had confirmed to them, for so many years now, by visual demonstrations. No one has been able to refute a sensory happening (observing movement, both to and fro, of the blood) with equally sensory observations, or to weaken by other experiments the results of experience adduced; on the contrary, there was not even any attempt made to provide opposing testimony by visual demonstration.

Meanwhile, there is no lack of those who, because of their inexperience and the roughness of their anatomical knowledge, have nothing to put against my concept of the circulation, but [nevertheless] cry out at it with empty and untrue assertions based on the authority of their teachers, or with some supposedly probable, empty sophisms. Others rail at it with a multitude of words, and those words not dignified but often abusive ones, even verging on wrangling and blows. With such these men merely draw attention to their emptiness, and sillinesses, and bad manners, and seem to expose their lack of arguments (which should be derived from sense), and to rave with false sophistic reason against sense. The waves of the Sicilian sea, stirred up by a storm, moan low as they are driven against the rocks inside Charybdis, and they break in pieces and are repelled in a mass of foam. Sense is equally the victor against mere sophistry.

If nothing could be admitted by sense without the evidence of reason, or on occasion against the dictate of reason, there would now be no problems for discussion. If faith through sense were not extremely sure, and stabilized by reasoning (as geometers are wont to find in their constructions), we would certainly admit no science: for geometry is a reasonable demonstration about sensibles from non-sensibles. According to its example, things abstruse and remote from sense become better known from more obvious and more noteworthy appearances. Aristotle advises us much better when, in discussing the generation of bees (*De generatione animalium*, Book 3, Chap. 10), he says: 'Faith is to be given to reason if the things which are being demonstrated agree with those which are perceived by sense: when they have become adequately known, then sense should be trusted more than reason'. Hence we ought to approve or disapprove or reject everything only after a very finely made examination. But to test and examine if things are rightly or wrongly spoken, ought to lead to sense, and to confirmation and establishment by the judgment of sense where nothing false will remain hidden. Whence Plato, in his *Critias*, states that it is [not] difficult to explain the things of which we shall be in a position to claim experience. And listeners who are devoid of experience are not fitted for science.

How hard and difficult it is to teach those who have no experience the things in which they lack such or have no sensible knowledge! And how unsuitable and hard to teach and inexperienced are they as listeners in respect of true science, obviously blind in respect to their judgments of colours and deaf in regard to those of harmonies! Who will ever teach blind people about the ebb and flow of the sea, or from a geometry diagram the sizes of the angles or the lengths of the sides? One inexperienced in things anatomical and (in so far as he does not grasp the matter with his own eyes and with his own concept therefrom deriving) to be regarded as par-blind in respect of them, is also unsuited for instruction. For he has no trained knowledge of the anatomist's subjects of discussion or of the natural sources from which he draws his proofs, but all things are equally unknown to him, both his facts and his inferences and his sources. For no knowledge can possibly come save from pre-existing knowledge, and this is one main reason why our knowledge about the heavenly bodies is so uncertain and conjectural. May I please learn from those, who claim smatterer-wise to know the causes and reasons of all things, how both eyes move simultaneously hither and thither and whither you will, and do not turn one at a time, that one thither and this one hither. Likewise both auricles of the heart, and so on. Because men do not know the causes of fevers or pestilence, or also the wonderful properties of some medicaments, and the reasons for such, should these for that reason be denied to the patient? Why is the foetus in the womb, not breathing air until the tenth month, not choked for lack of respiration? For when he is born in the seventh or eighth month, his respiration is inhibited soon after he takes his first breath, and he chokes for lack of air. Why still in his intra-uterine life or not yet having emerged from within the after-birth, will he have managed to retain life without respiration, while so soon as he has once been exposed to the air, he is unable to retain life unless he has breathed?

Because I see many held up and in doubt about the circulation, and some opposing it because they have not fully understood me, I will for their sake briefly recapitulate what I intended to say in my small book on the movement of the heart and blood. The blood contained in the veins and present in, so to speak, its reservoir where it is most abundant (that is, in the vena cava next the base of the heart and the right auricle), slowly growing warm from its internal heat and becoming more rarefied, swells up and rises in the way that fermenting things do. This dilates the auricle which, contracting with its pulsific faculty, drives the blood more frequently and more speedily into the right ventricle of the heart. This ventricle being filled, and subsequently by its systolic effort freeing itself of blood (since the tricuspid valves prevent regress into the auricle) drives the blood into the artery-like vein (where there is an open door) thereby distending it. Once in the artery-like vein and its branches, the blood is no longer able to move backwards because of the opposition of the sigmoid valves. At the same time the lungs, in turn extended and enlarged by inspiration and restricted by expiration, and their vessels similarly, show the blood this passage-way into the vein-like artery. From them the left auricle (dealing simultaneously, and equally with the right auricle, with movement, rhythm, order, and function) introduces the same blood into the left ventricle as does the right auricle into the right ventricle. Thence the left ventricle simultaneously and equally with the right (when a return to its place of origin is prevented by the hindrances raised by the resistant valves) drives the blood into the lumen of the aorta and consequently into all the branches of that artery. The arteries, filled by this sudden inthrust since they cannot equally suddenly relieve themselves of their extra content, are distended and forced more open and undergo diastole. Since the same procedure is continuously and constantly repeated, I conclude that the arteries, both in the lungs and elsewhere, would eventually become so distended and infarcted by so many heart-beats and drivings of blood into their cavities that either such indriving would altogether cease, or they would burst, or dilate so that they contained the whole mass of blood withdrawn from the veins unless they were relieved by an outflow of blood elsewhere.

The same reckoning holds about the ventricles of the heart when they are filled and, by the auricles, stuffed with blood. Unless the arteries emptied themselves to an equal extent, the ventricles would be at length maximally distended, and would remain devoid of any movement, and stationary. And this demonstrative conclusion of mine is both true and necessary, if the premises are true. Moreover, it is sense, not reason, which makes us surer, that is, seeing for ourselves, not stirring up the mind.

Moreover, I assert that the blood in the veins always runs everywhere from smaller into larger vessels, and hastens towards the heart from all the small parts. Whence I conclude that the amount which is continuously being introduced and which the arteries have received from the veins, reverts at length, and flows back to the source from which it was originally in course of being driven. In that way the blood moves in a circle, flowing from the heart through an impulse by the force of which it is driven through all the fibres of the arteries; thereafter; from all parts, in a continuation of the flow, it returns in succession through the veins, which absorb and remove it. Sense itself teaches that this is true, and the necessary conclusion from sensibles removes all occasion for doubting. Finally, this is what I shall attempt to explain and clarify by observations and experiments; I have not wanted to demonstrate from causes and probable beginnings but, through sense and experience, in anatomical fashion I have wished, as if by higher authority, to bring to confirmation.

From these things are to be noted what force and violence and upstirring of vehemence we perceive by touch and by sight in the heart and larger arteries, and I do not say that the systole and diastole of the pulse (in the larger and warmer animals) is the same in all the blood-containing vessels, or in all the blood-containing animals. It is, however, of such nature and size in all that a necessary consequence in a flow of blood and a more rapid course through the smaller arteries, the porosities of the parts, and the branches of all the veins. Hence the circulation.

For neither the smaller arteries nor the veins pulsate, but just the larger arteries and the ones nearer the heart in as much as they do not send out the blood as quickly as it is sent into them. You will be able to try with the artery dissected out and the blood leaping forth in full stream so that it gets out as easily as it comes in. In its artery of passage you will scarcely feel a pulse because, with an exit provided, the blood merely passes through without distending. In fishes, serpents, and colder-blooded animals the heart pulsates slowly and weakly so that even in the arteries you can scarcely feel a pulse, and it transmits the blood very slowly. Hence in these, as also in the smaller arterial fibres in man, there is no distinction of vessel coats or of blood, because they are not struck by the blood impulse.

In passing through a cut and opened artery the blood (as I have said) is neither impelling nor pulsatile. Hence it is clearly seen that the arteries do not undergo diastole through an innate pulsific faculty or through one transmitted to them by the heart, but solely by the impulse of the blood. For with it moving on in full flood, you will be able to see and feel by touch both systole and diastole, as I said before, and to recognize clearly all the differences of cardiac pulsation, rhythm and order, vehemence, and intermission in the outflow of fluid (like an image in a mirror). When water, by the strength and pressure of a siphon, is forced up through lead pipes, we can see and distinguish the individual compressions of the instrument (perhaps through considerable distances) in the very flow of the escaping water, also the order of the individual strokes, the beginning, increase, ending, and vehemence. So from the opening of the cut artery, where it is to be noted that, as in the case of the water, the outflow is continuous, although the jet now leaps out farther, now for a shorter distance. In arteries, apart from the shaking and the pulsation, or vibration (not equally discernible in all) of the blood, there is a continuous flow and movement occurring thence up to the point (namely, the right auricle) where the blood is back where it started.

All these things you can see in some fairly long artery, such as the carotid, that you have cut. You will be able to take it between your fingers and to regulate the outflow of blood, exploring as you wish the increase and decrease, and loss and recovery, of pulsation so that they are clearly discerned. And, while these things may become manifest in this way with the chest intact, you will also be able to experiment for a short while with the chest open and the lungs in consequence collapsed, and the movement of respiration lost. You will see, that is, contraction and emptying and paling of the left auricle and finally, in company with the left ventricle, its intermission and omission and abandoning of pulsation; and equally, from the opening in the cut artery, outflow of less and less blood in a thinner thread and with a weaker pulsation: and finally (with the blood supply and the left ventricular impulse failing) nothing further will emerge. You will be able to try the same with the artery-like vein ligated, and to take away the pulsation of the left auricle and restore it at will by removing the ligature. Hence the same thing is as clearly seen in this experiment as in moribund animals, namely, how first the left auricle would be desisting from movement and pulsation, thereafter the left ventricle, then the right ventricle, and finally the right auricle. So the point from which the vital faculty and pulsation first begin is also that at which they finally fail.

When these things are examined by sense, it is clear that the blood passes solely through the lungs (and not through the septum of the heart), and through them only when they are moved by respiration, not when they are collapsed and quiet. Whence it is probable why in the embryo (when it is not yet breathing) Nature opened the foramen ovale for the passage of the blood into the vein-like artery (where material for the left ventricle and auricle may be collected), an opening which she occludes in the young and in those breathing freely. It is also obvious why, when the vessels of the lung are overloaded and stuffed with blood, or in persons in whom the respiration is suffering from some fairly severe illness, the matter is so dangerous and a lethal sign. It is no less obvious why the lung blood is so redly glowing: for it is thinner as being filtered in these viscera. It is further to be noted, from the previously spoken epilogue from those who demand the causes of the circulation, and imagine the vigour of the heart to be the effector of all things, and (with Aristotle) believe it to be responsible not only for transmitting but also for attracting and generating blood; who believe also that the spirits and inflowing vital heat arise from the heart (and this by the innate heat of the heart, as if by the direct instrument of the psyche, or common bond, and prime organ for carrying out all the operations of life); who thus think that the blood and the movement of spirit, perfecting, and also warmth, are borrowed from the heart as from a source, also every property of the blood (which Aristotle says to be present in it as in hot water or boiling pottage) and that the heart is the prime cause of pulsation and life –. If I may speak openly, I do not think that these things are so (as they are commonly taken to be). There are also many things in the generation of the parts which encourage me towards the same view, but which it is not expedient to recite here. Shortly, perhaps, I shall publish things more wonderful than these, and likely to shed greater light on natural philosophy.

Meanwhile (with the kind permission of our learned men and a reverence for antiquity), I shall merely state and put forward without a demonstration the view that the heart, together with all the veins and arteries and the contained blood, is to be regarded as the beginning of the things that are in the body, the creator, fount and spring, and the prime cause of life. Just as the brain, with all its nerves, sensory organs, and spinal medulla included is (as they say) the one adequate organ of sense. But if by this term, 'the heart', they understand the body of the heart with its ventricles and auricles only, I do not believe that it is the fabricator of the blood (nor does the blood have force, vigour, reason, movement, or heat as the gift of the heart). Further, I do not think that diastole and distension have the same cause as systole and contraction, whether in the arteries or in the auricles or in the ventricles of the heart (but that part of the pulse which is called diastole has another cause different from that of systole, and should always everywhere precede each systole). And I think the prime cause of distension is the innate heat, and the prime distension is in the blood itself (in the manner of things fermenting, slowly attenuated, and swelling) and is extinguished last in the same. And I agree with Aristotle's likening it to the behaviour of pottage or of milk, in so far as a rise or fall of the blood does not come from vapours or exhalations or spirits, stirred up into some vaporous or aërial form, nor is it caused by an external agent, but it comes from an internal principle, the control exercised by Nature.

Nor is the heart, as some think, like a sort of burning coal or brazier or hot kettle, the source of heat and blood, but rather the blood, as being the warmest part of all in the body, gives to the heart (as to all the other parts) the heat which it has received. Thus the heart has assigned to it the coronary arteries and veins for the same purposes as vessels are assigned to the rest of the parts, namely, for the inflow of heat, its fomenting, and its preservation. All parts are warmer to the extent to which they consist more of blood, and, according to their greater richness in this fluid, they are said to be convertibly warmer. For this reason the heart, with its distinctive cavities, is deemed the warehouse, source, and permanent fireplace, not by reason of its fleshiness, but because of its blood content, like a hot kettle. In the same way as the liver, spleen, lungs, and other parts are considered hot because they possess many veins or blood-containing vessels. And in this way I assert the native heat, or innate warmth, to be the common instrument of all operations, and also the primary efficient cause of the pulse. This I do not as yet constantly assert, but merely propose as a thesis. I would gladly know what objections are raised against it, without verbal scurrility, railings, or abusive insults, by learned and honest men; and I shall be most grateful to whoever gives me such information.

There are thus, so to speak, parts and traces of the passage of the blood and of its circuit, namely, from the right auricle into the ventricle, from the ventricle through the lungs into the left auricle, thence through the left ventricle and into the aorta, and through all the arteries from the heart, through the porosities of the parts into the veins, and through the veins to the base of the heart, how quickly the blood returns!

By one experiment whoever wishes will be able to distinguish by means of veins. Let an arm be ligated (in the usual way) with a medium tight ligature, and let it remain ligated until, by movement of the arm, all the veins swell up exceedingly and the whole of the skin reddens markedly below the ligature. Then let the hand be plunged into very icy water or snow until the blood collecting below the ligature is sufficiently chilled. Next, with the ligature suddenly loosened, you will feel from the return of the cold blood how rapidly it hurries back to the heart, and what a change it makes in the heart on its return, so that it does not surprise you that some have fainted on release of the ligature after phlebotomy. This experiment shows that, below the ligature, the veins swell up not with thinned blood and inflated spirit or vapours (for the immersion into the cold would have depressed such bubbling out), but only with blood, and that blood such as cannot get back into arteries either through anastomoses or through blind wanderings. It also teaches how travellers through snow-clad mountains are often unexpectedly overcome by death; and many other such things.

Lest it seems difficult [to understand] how the blood can pass through all the pores of the parts and go in whatsoever direction it will, I will add one experiment. Those who are choked by a noose and those who are hanged by such have the same thing happen to them as happens to a ligated arm [see above]. That is to say, beyond the cord the face, eyes, lips, tongue, and all the upper parts of the head, are stuffed with very much blood, imbued with a maximum of red colour, and swollen to lividity. In such a body, after the noose has been loosened (in whatever position you have placed it), you will within not many hours see all the blood leave the face and head, and descend (as if carried down by its own weight) through the pores of the skin, flesh, and other parts from the supine and upper parts to the prone and lower ones. It fills especially all the lower parts and the skin, colouring all with black gore. Just as the blood is more lively and spirited in the living body and, with the porosities open, more penetrative than is dead and clotted blood, especially through a habit of body condensed by the cold of death, and with crowded and compressed passageways, so the route for the blood is much easier and readier through all parts in the living.

That very acute and ingenious man, René Descartes (to whom I am indebted for his honourable mention of my name), and others with himself, after removing a fish's heart and exposing it on a flat board, see it imitate a pulsation by drawing itself up. When it is erected, rises, and becomes strong, they assert that it is enlarging and opening out and that its ventricles are in consequence more capacious. According to my light, however, their observation is incorrect. For the heart is certainly contracted at that time, and all its capacities are rather in process of being constricted, and it is in its systole, not its diastole. It is not in its diastole and state of distension with its ventricles in consequence more capacious, when it is collapsing and relaxing in apparent weakness. But, as in death we do not say that the heart is in diastole, so do we talk about the relaxed, pre-systolic heart as being collapsed and devoid of all movement and rested, not as distended. For it is in course of being distended, and is properly speaking in its diastole when it is filled from the impulse of the blood through the contraction of the auricles, as is seen clearly enough in vivisections. It remains unknown, therefore, [to René Descartes] how far relaxation and relapse of the heart and arteries differ from distension or diastole; nor is he aware that the same thing is not the cause of distension, relaxation, and constriction. Rather are contrary effects due to contrary causes, and diverse movements due to diverse causes. So that all anatomists know well enough, that there are opposing antagonistic muscles of adduction and extension in each limb, and that for contrary and diverse movements contrary and diverse active organs have of necessity been fashioned by Nature. Nor am I in agreement with the view which he put forward, following Aristotle, of the efficient cause of pulsation being the same for systole and diastole, namely, effervescence or a sort of boiling up of the blood. For the movements in question are sudden strokes, and quick tappings. But nothing in fermentation or bubbling up rises and falls as if in the winking of an eye: there is merely a gentle sufflation and an adequate depression. This is apart from the fact that in vivisections it is possible to see for oneself the ventricles of the heart being distended and filled by the constriction of the auricles, and increasing in size according to the greater or lesser degree of their filling; and to note that distension of the heart is a certain violent movement brought about by an inthrust [of blood] and not by any attraction.

There are some who think that, just as food does not need any incitement for it to nourish plants, but is gradually attracted by the nearby small parts to the place of loss; so also in animals is no incitement necessary since the vegetative faculty carries out its work in similar fashion in animals and in plants. But the reason is in fact otherwise. Inflow of warmth is constantly required to keep the limbs of animals warm and, in the living, to conserve them with enlivening warmth and to restore the parts broken by injuries. But those are not needs so far as nutrition is concerned.

So much for the circulation! If it is either hindered or perverted or overstimulated, how many dangerous kinds of illness and surprising symptoms do not ensue? Either in veins, such as varices, abscesses, pains, haemorrhoids, and bleedings. Or in arteries, such as tumours, phlegmons, very intense and cutting pains, aneurysms, fleshy tumours, fluxions, sudden suffocations, asthma, stupor, apoplexies, and innumerable other things. Here is not the place for me to relate how quickly and when, like a charm, certain otherwise irremediable troubles are removed and cured. In my medical observations and in my pathology I shall be able to tell of things which have not hitherto been observed by anyone.

In order that I may make your satisfaction more complete, learned Riolan, seeing that you do not believe in the occurence of a circulation in the mesenteric veins, try this simple experiment. In a vivisection, ligate the portal vein near the visceral part of the liver. You will see, from the swelling up of the veins below the ligature, that the same thing is happening as occurs in the administration of a phlebotomy from the placing of a ligature on the arm, revealing the passage of the blood at that point. And, as you appear to think that the blood can go back from the veins into the arteries through anastomoses, ligate the vena magna descendens, in a vivisection, next the bifurcation of the femoral veins. Then, once an exit is given by cutting some artery, you will see the whole mass of blood withdrawn in a short bout of cardiac pulsation from all the veins (even including the ascending vena cava) but beyond the ligature the femoral veins (their lower parts at least) remaining full. Which could in no wise come to pass had the blood been able to get back anywhere into the arteries through anastomoses.

THE FIRST LETTER OF WILLIAM HARVEY IN THE 1651–1657 SERIES. TO PAUL MARQUARD SCHLEGEL, OF HAMBURG

For my part I congratulate you, learned Sir, on the remarkable dissertation with which you have recently made reply to (as you say) your erstwhile teacher, the famous anatomist, Riolan. For truth, unconquered ever, has shown how the pupil can overcome the master. I myself was getting a sponge ready for his latest arguments, but being [more] directly intent on my essays on the generation of animals (which have just been published and of which I send you a copy). I have not yet found it convenient to use [the instrument in question]. And, indeed, I rejoice because my silence (as I learn from your postscript) has evoked your very lucid thoughts for the common benefit of learned men. For I see clearly that by your most exquisite little book (which I am not unduly praising by referring to it in such terms) you have skilfully and vigorously confuted all Riolan's attacks on my earlier statement about the circulation and have upset the supports of his own more recent view. So that I need not labour excessively about any further reply. Very many points could indeed be raised in support of the truth, and some of them such as throw further light on the art of medicine. But of those we shall perhaps get a glimpse later.

Meanwhile, as Riolan exerts himself to the utmost to deny a passage of blood through the lungs to the left ventricle of the heart and makes it all go thither through the septum; as by the same token he boasts that the basis of the Harveian circulation is going to be completely upset (though I have never set that feature up as the basis of my circulation. For a circuit of the blood occurs in very many blood-containing animals in which you will find no lungs), I have pleasure in describing here an experiment, tried out recently by myself in the presence of several colleagues, and from the implications of which there is no escape. The artery-like vein and the vein-like artery and the aorta were ligated in the cadaver of a throttled human being, and the left ventricle of the heart was opened. I then introduced a small tube through the vena cava into the right ventricle and at the same time fastened on to the tube an ox's bladder as is usually done in the injection of clysters. This I filled almost full of warm water, and injected it with great force into the ventricle mentioned so that almost a pound of fluid passed over into it and its neighbouring auricle. What happened? The ventricle in question (together with its auricle) swelled up violently, but not even a small drop of water or of blood escaped through the gap in the left ventricle. When the aforementioned ligatures had been released, the same tube was introduced into the artery-like vein, and after a tight ligature had been made to prevent the water from getting back into the right ventricle, I attempted to drive this water into the lungs. At once it shot forward, mixed with a large amount of blood, from the cut in the left ventricle in such a way that as much water came out from the cut in question as was pushed into the lungs at the individual compressions of the bladder. You can try it so often as you wish and discover that it is so.

With this one experiment you will easily have silenced all Riolan's arguments about this matter. He has, however, relied so much on such arguments that, without experimental support, he has decided to invent a new circulation; indeed, he has stated that, unless the old doctrine of the circulation is overthrown, his own cannot be established. The great man must be pardoned for not having been the first to discover a truth hidden in a secret place. But that he, so skilled in things anatomical as he is, so strongly opposes a truth lighted up by the clearest rays of reason, is at least evidence of envy (to say nothing worse). But perhaps even Riolan should be excused on the ground that he has written those things not as representing his personal view, but officially and in his desire to deserve well of his colleagues. It was doubtless fitting for the Dean of the College of Paris to keep Galen's medicine in good repair, and to allow no innovations to enter his school without the fullest airing lest (as he says) the precepts and dogmata of the physicians be disturbed, and lest the pathology which has obtained for so many years, with the agreement of the physicians, in assigning the causes of diseases, be corrupted. He has accordingly acted the part of the orator rather than that of the skilled anatomist. As Aristotle warns us, it is as absurd to expect demonstrative proofs from the orator as it is to expect persuasive

ones from the demonstrator or teacher. However, for the sake of
the old friendship existing between us and for the high praises
which he bestowed on my doctrine of the circulation, I cannot
regard it as fitting to say anything harsh against Riolan.

I come back, therefore, to yourself, learned Schlegel, and I do
really wish that I had more fully and more clearly explained to you
what I said about anastomosis in my dissertations to Riolan, so
that you had had no doubt at all from that source. And I could
wish you had also taken into account not only what I had there
denied, but also what I there asserted (about the transfer of blood
from the arteries into the veins), especially as in those passages I
seem to have indicated some reason for my statement and my
denial. I said indeed, I confess (and I even now assert), that I had
never found visible anastomoses. But that had been particularly
said against Riolan, who postulated a circulation of the blood in
the larger vessels only. With these vessels, therefore, anastomoses
(if any existed) should have been made conformable, that is to say,
rather large, and visible. Although, therefore, it is true that I
totally deny anastomoses[1] are found anywhere as such as
commonly understood and as they have been handed down from
Galen's time (namely, as openings of veins and of arteries
mutually inosculating), I have nevertheless in the same dissertation confessed that I have discovered their equivalent in three
places, namely, in the cerebral plexus, in the spermatic preparative arteries and veins, and in the umbilical arteries and veins. I
shall now, therefore, reveal at greater length of your sake, learned
Sir, why I denied the common anastomoses, and what is my guess
about the passage of blood from arterioles into venules.

All reasonable physicians of past and recent times have believed
that there exists a sort of mutual exchange, or advance and
recession, of blood between veins and arteries, and because of
such belief have imagined anastomoses of varying degrees of
invisibility (that is, certain inconspicuous openings or hidden
foramina) through which the blood flowed in both directions and
migrated out from vessel into vessel and back again. On that
account it is not to be wondered at if Riolan has discovered
somewhere among the ancients something which appears to
harmonize with the doctrine of the circulation of the blood. For a
circulation of that sort teaches nothing other than that the blood

[1]Granted I have used the term 'anastomosis' for the opening of vessels.

flows unceasingly from veins into arteries and back again from arteries into veins. Because, however, those ancients thought that this movement took place indeterminately, and as if haphazardly, in one and the same place, and through the same channels, I imagine that they coined the expression 'anastomoses' (that is, mutual inosculations serving both sets of vessels). However, the circulation which I discovered teaches clearly that a forward and backward flow of blood must take place, and that at different times and places, and through other and other channels and pathways; determinately also, and with some objective in view, the parts being constructed for that purpose with extreme foresight and wonderful skill. So that the doctrine of the movement of blood from the veins into the arteries and from the latter back into the former (which antiquity understood only with a slight degree of conjecture, and which it also drew up in confused and disordered fashion) appears, after I have laid down definite and necessary causes, extremely clear, orderly, and very true. And thence it came about that, since I saw blood passing from the veins into the arteries by way of the heart with great artifice and a very fine provision of valves, I thought that the same blood could not return to the veins from the arteries without an equally wonderful device (wherever there is no transudation through the pores of the flesh). Accordingly, I deservedly suspected the anastomoses of the ancients because such never come to our visual notice, nor does reason persuade us that any such things should be accepted. Because, therefore, in those three places (which I have just mentioned) I find a transfer from arteries into veins equivalent to the anastomosis of the ancients, and it is an even better guarantee that blood transferred from the arteries into the veins cannot run the opposite way back into the former, and since a device of that sort is more elaborate, and more suitable for the circulation of the blood, I have therefore considered that those anastomoses invented by the ancients should be rejected. But, you ask, what then is this device? And what are those channels? Doubtless arterioles, which are always considerably smaller, perhaps twice or three times so, than the veins which they accompany and slowly approach, and within the coats of which they finally disappear. And I could therefore have believed that the blood brought forward through these vessels proceeded for a short distance between the coats of the veins; and that there the same thing happened as comes about at the junction of the ureters with the bladder and of the bile duct with the duodenum. For the ureters insinuate themselves obliquely and tortuously into the coats of the bladder so that in no way do they reproduce the character of anastomoses; sometimes, however, they afford passage to calculi, pus, and blood. Through them you will readily fill the bladder with air or water, but by no effort may you force anything back from the bladder into the ureter. I am not, however, concerned about the etymology of the word, for I do not believe it to be advantageous to philosophic principle to decide something about the works of Nature from the meaning of words, or to summon anatomical disputes before the grammatical tribunal. For it is not so much a matter of asking what words properly mean as it is of asking how they are ordinarily used. For custom is of the greatest importance not only in many other matters, but especially so in respect of the meaning of words. For this reason I consider that we should definitely avoid using unaccustomed words, or ones which though common have been used over-long in a sense other than that which is apt for our purpose. You counsel well indeed, but who can understand the matter, call it what he will? Since, however, it has hitherto been rather incorrectly explained (as will be shown by the things I have to say farther on), and as I think an old name is not well suited to a new thing, and often makes for mind-wandering in those you wish to teach, I agree that there exists a passage from arteries into veins, and that on occasion directly and without the intervention of fleshy substance. It does not, however, occur in the way that it has been believed to do, and as you yourself meant where you say that, strictly speaking, anastomoses rather than an anastomosis are needed, that is to say, in order that vessels may open equally on both sides so that blood may freely pass on this side and on that. And hence it comes about that you would less correctly solve that doubtful point, namely, why, with arteries and veins lying equally open, the blood nevertheless sets its course from the former into the latter, but never in turn from the latter into the former. For what you say of the drive of blood through the arteries does not completely remove the difficulty attached to this matter. If in a live animal you ligate the aorta near the left ventricle of the heart, and draw off all the blood from the arteries, the veins on the other hand are meanwhile visibly full of blood, so that it neither flows back spontaneously into the arteries nor can it be forcibly pushed back into them, though even in the dead animal it spontaneously flows down through the very narrow pores of the flesh and skin from the upper to the lower parts. The passage of the blood across into the veins is indeed effected by that drive, and not by any dilatation of the veins drawing blood into them like bellows. There are not, however, any vascular anastomoses by copulation such as you say occur, namely, those in which vessels are mutually opposed little mouth to little mouth. There is merely an opening of an artery into a vein in exactly the same way as we noted about the insertion of the ureters into the bladder (and of the bile duct into the duodenum). The urine is freely driven from the ureters into the bladder, but all back flow from the bladder into the ureters is prevented; nay, indeed, the more are the sides of the ureters compressed and ascent of urine into them prevented. And from this hypothesis the cause of that experiment which I have just mentioned is readily given. I add that I am quite unable to admit anastomoses of the kind usually imagined because, as the artery is much smaller than the vein, the walls of the two vessels cannot mutually join in such a way as to make a common passage. To be so joined they must be of equal magnitude. Moreover, those vessels (where they terminate), after making a circuit, must encounter each other, not however (as it happens) reach straight to the extremities of the body. And for their part the veins, if they joined the arteries in mutual embraces, would necessarily pulsate because of the continuity of the parts.

So that I may at last make an ending, I say that, though I judge the industry of everyone to be praiseworthy, I do not ever remember praising my own. However, you, I think, most distinguished Sir, deserve very great praise for the hard work involved in your disquisition on the ox' liver and for the judgment displayed in your observations. Continue (as you are doing) to ornament the republic of letters with the gifts of your talent. For thus will you put in your debt all other learned men and most of all

Your affectionate

WILLIAM HARVEY

Given in London, this 26th day of March, 1651.

THE first of the eight letters was given in London on 26 March, 1651, and was directed to Paul Marquard Schlegel, of Hamburg, a very strong supporter of Harvey's views on the circulation. Schlegel had been born in

Hamburg on 23 August, 1605, and had taken up the study of natural and medical sciences against the wishes of his father, a prosperous merchant of that city. He had begun such work in Altdorf in 1626, but later had moved to Wittenberg, where he was attached to his later to be famous fellow-countryman, Werner Rolfinck (1599–1673); when in 1629 the latter had become Professor of Anatomy and Botany in Jena, Schlegel had followed him thither. In 1631 he undertook a scientific journey which in the event lasted some years, Holland and England being the first two countries visited. From England he had gone to France, whence after a fairly long stay in Paris, Lyon, and Montpellier he had moved on to Italy. After visiting Rome and Naples he had returned home to Germany, where he at once became Professor of Botany, Anatomy, and Surgery in Jena. In 1642 he was called to Hamburg to be Chief Physician there. He died on 20 February, 1653. In 1650, at Hamburg, he had produced *De sanguinis motu commentatio, in qua praecipue in Joannis Riolani sententiam inquiritur*. This publication is well worth reading; in it Schlegel attacked the ideas of his former teacher, Jean Riolan, jr., about the functions of the portal vein. The finding on a throttled man which is mentioned in the second paragraph of Harvey's letter to Schlegel is an important piece in the total circulatory story told by the former.

THE SECOND LETTER TO THE EXCELLENT GIOVANNI NARDI, OF FLORENCE

I should have written to you long ago, but in part public troubles did not permit, in part getting ready for the press my book on the generation of animals delayed my writing. For, as one who had received from you not only books (on the outstanding repute of which I congratulate you very much and warmly) but also very kind letters, I did not think it very fair to reply to so distinguished a person with just a miserable little letter. I have therefore written to-day so that you may know that I value very highly your repute and good will, and store up in the depths of my mind memories of your friendly offices to me in Florence (and to my nephew when he was busy there). I should like, illustrious Sir, to learn without delay what you are doing and what are your feelings about this work of mine. For I care not at all for the judgments and censures of the smatterers, whose mind also is not dexterous in judging, and who are wont to praise nothing save that which they have themselves accomplished. So soon as I learn that you will survive and remain mindful of me, I shall enjoy more often such literary exchange, and see that other books are sent off to you.

I wish your most serene Duke many prosperous years, and you yourself happy living.

Farewell, learned Sir,

Yours always

WILLIAM HARVEY

London, 15 July, 1651.

THE second, fourth, and seventh of the letters of Harvey were sent to Doctor Giovanni Nardi, a literary and medical Florentine friend who was responsible for, *inter alia*, a new edition of Lucretius.

THE THIRD LETTER IN REPLY TO ROBERT MORISON, M.D., OF PARIS

Distinguished Sir!

The reason why I have not up to now replied at all to your very kind letters is because the small book of M. Pecquet (on which you were seeking my opinion) did not reach my hands until towards the end of last month. It was being held up, I believe, by someone who either through neglect in delivering it, or through eagerness to peruse the new literature, prevented me that long from enjoying it. So, therefore, that you may know clearly my feeling about this work, I am definitely very full of praise for the author's diligence in the dissection of cadavers, for his dexterity in contriving fresh experiments, and for his shrewdness in judging them. It is indeed a difficult path we tread to the hidden things of truth, and by relying on the findings of our senses we acknowledge God as our guide in relation to His own works and as our instructor about them, while that specious way, which blinds by the mere dazzle of syllogisms, leads for the most part into the wilderness, and exhibits only a probable and very largely sophistical conjecture about things.

Indeed, I even congratulate myself that Pecquet has confirmed my view about the circulation of the blood by such sure experiments and clear reasonings. I could, however, wish that he had noticed one thing, namely, that the heart indulges in a triple kind of movement, to wit, a systole in which it contracts and expels the blood contained within itself; then a sort of relaxation, the opposite of the previous movement, by which the cardiac fibres given over to movement are slackened, and these two movements are in the very substance of the heart, as they are also in all other muscles. Finally there is diastole, in which the heart is distended by the blood driven out of its auricles into its ventricles; and the ventricles, filled and distended in this way, excite the heart to contract: and this movement always precedes the systole which is immediately to succeed it.

With regard to the lacteal veins discovered by Aselli, and the further careful work of Pecquet through which he found the receptaculum or cisterna chyli, a receiver and distributor of chyle, and the small channels leading thence into the subclavian veins, I will tell you freely (since you so request) my feeling on the matter. Long ago, indeed (may I venture to say) before Aselli was in process of publishing his little book, I had looked carefully at those little white channels, and the amount of milk in the several parts of the body, and particularly in the glands of younger animals (in the mesentery they are in particularly great number), and it was through that, I thought, that the thymus in the calf and the lamb came to taste so pleasant, and to be called by our countryfolk (in the vernacular) *the sweet bread*. However, for very many reasons, and because of various experiments, it has never been possible to induce me to believe that that milky fluid is chyle, being carried that way from the intestines to all parts of the body for their nourishment. I have rather believed that it happens occasionally by chance, and proceeds from too rich a suckling and excellence of concoction; that is, by the same law of Nature which is responsible for producing fat, marrow, semen, abundance of hair, and the rest. And, just as pus is formed in the due digestion of ulcers and wounds, and the nearer it comes to the consistency of milk, that is, according as it becomes whiter, smoother, and more homogeneous, so is it considered more laudable, and therefore some of the ancients thought milk itself to be akin to pus. Though, therefore, there would be no question about the existence of those vessels, I cannot agree with Aselli that they are chyliferous, and that especially for the reasons I must now mention, which lead my mind to the opposite conclusion. The fluid contained in the lacteal veins seems to be perfectly pure milk such as is found in the lacteal veins of the mammae. However, it seems to me to be unlikely (Auzout, in the letter he wrote to Pecquet, seems equally doubtful) that the milk is chyle, and so the whole body is nourished on milk. The reasons adduced to the contrary to prove that it is chyle are not strong enough to convince me. I shall, therefore, wish first to have it demonstrated to me by definite forces of reasons and clear-cut experiments that it is indisputably chyle which, carried that way from the intestines, supplies aliment for the body as a whole. For, unless there is first agreement on this matter, all the care spent on further investigation and more painstaking inquiry into the nature of those things will be fruitless so far as I am concerned. Moreover, how can these ducts help in carrying round the chyle as a whole, or the nutriment of the body, if they are seen to differ in different animals? In some they go off to the liver, in others only to the porta hepatis, in others again they reach neither point. In certain animals, a large number of them are visible in the pancreas; in other animals, the thymus abounds with them; in some animals, however, you will see none of them in either of these organs. Indeed, in very many animals chyle-conveying channels of that sort are not found at all (Licetus, Letter XVI, p. 83; Sennert, Practice, Book 5, Section 1, Part 3, Chap. 2): and they do not occur all the time in any, although vessels destined for nutrition must necessarily be present in all animals all the time: because the loss inflicted by outflow of spirits and of body components can only be restored by constant nourishment of the same parts. In addition, the narrowness and lack of capacity of these vessels seems to render them as inadequate for the suggested purpose as their structure makes them unsuited for it. For the smaller branchlets ought to end in larger ones, and these latter should similarly terminate in others more capacious, and at length finish as a very large trunk, corresponding in amplitude to all the other channels put together, just as is to be seen in the portal vein and its branchlets, and as the trunk of a tree is equal to its roots. So, if the channels carrying some fluid towards a destination ought to equal in greatness those carrying the same fluid away from it, then the chyliferous ducts (which Pecquet locates in the thorax) should correspond in capacity to at least both ureters. For otherwise those who drink a gallon and more of mineral waters could not in so short a time pass them on through these vessels into the bladder. And indeed, when the matter of the urine passes in quantity by those routes, I do not see how those veins can keep their milky colour and meanwhile the urine from them be quite untinged by their whiteness. For I add that the chyle is not in all animals, nor all the time, of the same consistency and colour as milk, and in consequence, if those vessels carried chyle, they could not always (though, however, they do in fact do so) contain a white fluid, but they would from time to time be tinged yellow or green or some other colour according as urines take on different colours from the eating of rhubarb, asparagus, Indian fig, and the rest, and when filled full of clear mineral waters would show no colour at all. Moreover, if that white matter passed from the intestines into those ducts or was attracted by the same, that kind of fluid should certainly be discoverable somewhere in the intestines themselves, or in their spongy coats. For it does not seem probable that a fluid, by a simple and sudden filtration through the intestine, takes on another nature and forms milk. Indeed, if the chyle were merely filtered through the coats of the intestines, it should surely retain some trace of its original nature, and resemble in colour and odour the fluid found in the intestines, and indeed smell offensively. For whatever is contained in the intestines from top to bottom is tinged with bile, and smells noxious. And because of that some think that the body is nourished by chyle thinned out to vapour. Since vapours exhaling from even foetid matters in a still often do not smell badly.

M. Pecquet attributes the cause of movement of this milky fluid to respiration. For my part, though there are many things to persuade me to the contrary, I will nevertheless say nothing about that matter until he has privately decided the nature of the liquid. If, however, I may grant (what he asks to have given him, though he has not succeeded in proving his right to it by any force of argument), that the chyle is continuously carried away by that path, that is to say, is led off from the intestines to the subclavian veins, in which the vessels recently discovered by him end; I should certainly have to say that the chyle before reaching the heart mixes with the blood which will soon be entering the right ventricle of the heart to obtain there a richer concoction. Moreover, why may they not equally justly say that the same chyle passes into the porta hepatis, and thence into the liver and into the cava? As it is said to have been seen to do by Aselli and others. Indeed, why may we not equally well believe that the chyle enters the farthest openings of the mesenteric veins and thereby mixes at once with the blood, so that it gets concoction and perfecting from the blood's heat, and serves for the nourishment of the parts as a whole? For indeed the heart becomes more highly esteemed than the other parts, and can be called the source of heat and of life, only in so far as it contains the most blood within itself. This blood it holds not in veins as do other parts, but in a roomy sinus, as in a reservoir. That it is so is in my view proved by the fact that the provision of arteries and veins to the intestines is so rich, greater indeed than to any part of the body as a whole in the same way as the pregnant uterus abounds in so very great a supply of vessels. For Nature never does anything thoughtlessly. And hence all blood-carrying animals which require nourishment are provided with mesenteric veins, but only a very few with lacteal veins, and the provision of those is inconstant. Wherefore, if I am to judge of the use of parts as I see them commonly in the majority of animals, those white threads very like spiders' webs have definitely not been instituted for the transport of nourishment. Nor should the fluid discernible within them be called by the name, 'chyle'. But rather is it the mesenteric vessels which are destined for that function. For from the substance of which it consists an animal must of necessity grow and in consequence be nourished, one and the same substance causing its nourishment and its increase. And in consequence an animal increases naturally according as nutriment has become immediately available to it from the beginning. It is, moreover, a most definite fact (as I have said elsewhere) that the embryos of all blood-carrying animals are nourished by the mother by the help of the umbilical vessels, that is to say, by means of the circulation. They are not, however, nourished directly by the blood as most people believe, but in the way that is customary among feathered creatures, who live first on albumen and yelk, which is finally drawn up into and occluded by the abdomen of the chick. Moreover, all the umbilical vessels are inserted into the liver, or at least pass through it, even in those animals the umbilical vessels of which are inserted into the portal vein, just as in chicks the vessels coming from the yelk always end there. As, therefore, the chick is fed on a previously prepared source of nourishment (namely, albumen and yelk), so in exactly the same way it is nourished for the whole course of its life. And it happens similarly (as I have elsewhere stated) to all embryos, namely, that the aliment, mixed with blood, is carried through their veins and at last reaches the heart. Thence it passes out again through the arteries and off to all parts of the body as a whole. The post-natal foetus, now independent and no longer relying on its mother for nutrition, uses its own stomach and intestines just as the chick makes use of the egg or plants of the soil to draw concocted nourishment therefrom. For just as the chick at the beginning, by means of the circulation, was seeking its food from the egg by means of the umbilical vessels (arteries and veins), so later on, after being hatched, it is nourished through the mesenteric veins from the intestines. In both cases, therefore, chyle is passing through the liver in the same way and by the same channels. Nor do I see any reason against the passage of the chyle in all animals by the same route as it is carried in a particular one. Nor indeed, if a circuit of the blood is necessary (as in fact it is) for this purpose, can you devise any other way?

I praise very highly the industry of M. Pecquet, and the reservoir discovered by him. It does not, however, impress me so greatly as to divert me from the view which I have just enounced. For I have often discovered different receptacles for milk in young animals, and in the human embryo I have found the thymus so swollen with the fluid that at first glance I suspected an abscess and believed the lungs to be in a state of suppuration, for the swelling appeared larger than the lungs themselves. And often I have found abundance of milk in the nipples of newborn infants, as also in the breasts of corpulent and over-fat young men. I have also seen in a fat and bulky deer a receptacle full of milk of such size that it could readily have been compared with an abomasum: it was in evidence at the spot where Pecquet located his cistern.

These are the points, learned Sir, which I should at present mention in a reply to your letter. For the rest, if you will offer my very best wishes to M. Pecquet and M. Gayant, your good health will be the wish of

Yours affectionately and respectfully

WILLIAM HARVEY

Given in London
the 28 April, 1652.

DR. ROBERT MORISON (1620–83), of Paris, to whom the third of the eight letters was sent by Harvey, was, according to the *D.N.B.*, M.A., Ph.D. (Aberdeen) at twenty, but, after bearing arms in the Royalist cause, went to Paris and later became a physician and botanist and got to know Charles II, whom he accompanied to England at the Restoration, and by whom he was appointed his Senior Physician, King's Botanist, and Superintendent of all the royal gardens. The rest of his life was botanical and medical, in Oxford.

Harvey's letter to Morison necessitates a word or two about the lacteals and thoracic duct, and about Gasparo Aselli (1581–1626) and Jean Pecquet (1622–74). Aselli discovered the lacteals in 1622, but did not publish his finding until 1627, i.e. posthumously, and erred in making his 'lacteal veins' end in the liver. Jean Pecquet, while a student in the University of Montpellier, discovered the thoracic duct in 1647 in an animal opened during digestion, and in many experiments traced it downwards and discovered its origin in the receptaculum chyli, into which the lacteals empty. Tracing it in the other direction, he found its termination in the subclavian vein. He published in 1651, and Van Horne, who had been working independently of Pecquet, corroborated his findings in 1652.

THE FOURTH LETTER TO THE EXCELLENT AND LEARNED DOCTOR GIOVANNI NARDI, OF FLORENCE

Famous and distinguished Sir!

It certainly gave me the greatest pleasure when your letter recently reached me and at the same time your learned comments on Lucretius, for I saw both that you were still alive and also that you were busy with the inner rites of Phoebus Apollo. It was certainly a cause of rejoicing to me that very learned men here and there were advancing the republic of letters even in this age, in which the crowd of writers devoid of taste is as numerous as a swarm of flies on a very hot day, and we are almost stifled by the stench of their thin and trifling productions. There were several things which I was very pleased to read in your book, and it was a joy to see that you had attributed almost the same efficient cause to plague as I had ascribed to the generation of animals. It is however, difficult to explain how the idea, or form, or vital principle, can be carried across from the genitor to the genetrix, and thence into the conceptus or ovum, and thence again into the foetus; and in this last reproduce not only the genitor's own likeness or external appearance, but also chance peculiarities, such as character, faults, inherited diseases, scars, and moles. All these are inherent in the geniture and semen and accompany that specific property (by whatever name it is to be called), from which not only is the animal established, but also by which it is governed and preserved to the last end of life. While, I say, those things are not easy to put into words, yet I think it is equally difficult to understand how the essence of a pestilence or of leprosy can be communicated even to a distance by contact, especially through an intermediary such as by the agency of woollen or linen clothes, or other familiar furnishing, or even by means of walls, stone, rubble, and the rest, as in Leviticus, Chap. 14, it is held to happen. How, I ask, can contagion long dormant in things of that kind, later emerge from them and that after a long interval, and produce something similar to itself even in another body? And that not in one or two only, but in many and without reference to strength, sex, age, temperature, or mode of living, and meanwhile so fatally to this same point that the evil can by no art be kept at a distance or immediately be averted. For assuredly it does not seem less probable for the form or vital principle or idea (whether substantive or chance) to be so transferred into something else that at length an animal is produced as if on purpose and with design, with foresight, intellect, and divine art.

These are among the more hidden matters, learned Nardi, and they call for your shrewd attention. Nor is there any reason for you to plead advancing years, for I am myself now almost an octogeniarian and, although my physical powers are tottering with my body broken, yet with my mind active I give myself up most gladly to studies of this sort. I send to you with this letter three books on the subject about which you were asking me. Further, if in my name you will thank the Duke of Tuscany most warmly for the unusual honour which he once did me when I was in Florence, and will offer him my good wishes for his safety and prosperity, you will be doing a most kind thing to

Your devoted and affectionate

WILLIAM HARVEY

Given in London,
30 November, 1653.

THE FIFTH LETTER TO JOHANN DANIEL HORST, CHIEF PHYSICIAN OF HESSE-DARMSTADT

Excellent Sir!

I congratulate myself very much that, after so long a lapse of time and despite such a separation in space, you have not lost me from your memory, and I could wish that it might be given to me to satisfy your request in the way that you would like. But in fact my age denies me that pleasure, partly because I have not many more years to go, partly because I am often unduly distressed by recurrence of ill health. With regard to Riolan's opinion and his view about the circulation of the blood, he has very obviously achieved mighty trifles by great effort and I cannot see that his fictions have brought pleasure to anyone. Schlegel wrote more carefully and modestly and, had the fates permitted, would doubtless have taken the force out of Riolan's arguments and even out of his taunts. But I learn, and that with sorrow, that he shuffled off this mortal coil of ours a few months since. Moreover, the things you ask me about the lacteal veins and the so-called thoracic ducts demand sharp-sighted eyes and a mind free from other cares in order that you can establish anything definite about those very small vessels; to me, however, as I have said, neither of the prerequisites mentioned is any longer available. About two years ago, when asked my view on this matter, I replied at some length to the effect that it was not sufficiently clear whether the fluid was chyle, or a constituent of milk soon about to turn into fat, which passes through those white vessels: further, that the vessels in question are lacking from certain animals, for instance, from birds and fishes. As, however, the standard of nutrition of such animals is probably identical with that of quadrupeds, and no sufficient reason can be assigned why in the embryo all food material is carried through the umbilical vein across the liver, but that no longer happens after the foetus has become independent and escaped from the confine of the womb. As, moreover, the thoracic ducts are over-small, and the foramen (through which the chyle passes into the subclavian vein) is too narrow for all the produce which is to suffice for the body as a whole to be able to pass that way, I also asked why so immense a number of arteries and veins is supplied to the intestines if nothing is to be carried away from them, especially as they are membranous parts and therefore need less by way of a blood supply.

These and other observations of the same sort I have already put on record, not because I am stubbornly addicted to the view in question, but so that I can find out what can be said against it by the supporters of the new view. I praise highly the singular industry of Pecquet and of others in searching into the truth. Nor do I doubt but that many things have been buried to date in the well of Democritus which are destined to be disclosed by the tireless diligence of the succeeding age. These things I had to write in reply to you in the circumstances, and you, I hope, will with your singular humanity take them in good part. Farewell, learned Sir, and live happily. As your

heartily devoted

WILLIAM HARVEY wishes that you may!

London, 1 February, 1654-5.

THE SIXTH LETTER TO THE DISTINGUISHED AND EMINENT GENTLEMAN, JOHANN DANIEL HORST, CHIEF PHYSICIAN OF HESSE-DARMSTADT

Excellent Sir!

My now too long a tale of years causes me to repress from sheer weariness any desire to explore new subtleties, and after long labours my mind is too fond of peace and quiet for me to let myself become too deeply involved in an arduous discussion of recent discoveries. So I am far from setting myself up as a suitable mediator in this dispute. It was with a desire to gratify you that I recently rewrote, in reply to your inquiry about my view on the lacteal veins and thoracic ducts, the answers I had earlier made to a certain physician of Paris. Not indeed because I was certain of the correctness of the view I advanced, but so that I might with those various objections twist a little the ears of those who think that they have revealed all on the basis of a very few discoveries only.

With regard to your answering letter, however, I did not attribute to chance the collection of that milky fluid in the vessels of Aselli, as if it were without definite causes for its existence, but I did say that it is not found in all animals at all time (as a uniform process of nutrition seems to demand). Nor is it necessary that a material which is already thin and rather dilute and is about to end, after further concoction, in fat shall solidify in the dead animal. I brought forward the case of pus only outside the direct line of argument. Indeed, the main pivot of our debate had lain in the fact that the fluid which is contained in Aselli's lacteals is clearly chyle. This I certainly do not think you demonstrate by the liquid, while you say that chyle must be drawn off from the intestines but cannot be carried from them in any way by means of arteries, veins, or nerves so that it remains for that office to be performed by the help of the lacteals. I myself indeed see no serious reason why the innumerable veins, which everywhere worm through the intestines and carry back to the heart the blood received in those parts from the arteries, cannot simultaneously suck up the chyle penetrating into those regions and carry it to the heart and this the rather because some chyle probably goes straight from the stomach before reaching the intestines, though no lacteals are distributed to the stomach. For how otherwise account for the rapid recovery of spirits and strength in cases of fainting?

With regard to the things which you say you have written to Bartholin, I have no doubt that he will reply to the same as you desire, and there is no need for me to trouble you further in the matter. I will only say (keeping quiet about other paths) that the nutritious juice can as readily be carried by the uterine arteries and distil into the uterus as serum can pass through the renal arteries into the kidneys. And that juice cannot be called preternatural; neither ought it to be compared with the vagitus uterinus, as the juice is always present in pregnant women while the vagitus occurs extremely seldom. With regard to what you go on to add, namely, that the excreta of the newborn differ from the excreta of those who have even once partaken of milk, I for my part admit practically no difference between them save in colour, and I think that the blackness of the faeces may rightly be ascribed to their long stay in the bowel.

As to your suggestion that I should deal with the true use of the newly-discovered ducts, that is indeed a matter of greater moment than befits a broken old man entangled in other cares. Nor can such a task conveniently be entrusted to many, even supposing the helps you mention were at hand. However, they are not so, and Highmore does not live in this part, nor have I seen him over seven years. I had these things to write at the present. Do you, distinguished Sir, deem them friendly and well-wishing, as coming from

Yours affectionately and respectfully,

WILLIAM HARVEY

London, 13 July, 1655 (O.S.).

THE addressee of the fifth and sixth of the Harvey letters had been born at Giessen in 1616, and became Professor and Court Physician there in 1637; he was to die in 1685.

The well of Democritus in the fifth letter refers to truth being sunk in it, e.g. in Diogenes Laertius, *Lives of Eminent Philosophers*, Book IX, Pyrrho, Section 72, translated by R. D. Hicks in the Loeb Classical Library, 1931, there is a passage which reads, 'Furthermore, they find Xenophanes, Zeno of Elea, and Democritus to be sceptics . . . Democritus because he rejects qualities, saying . . . "Of truth we know nothing, for truth is in a well".' A note at the foot of the page says that 'This proverbial expression is inadequate; a more literal rendering of ἐν βύθῳ would be "in an abyss"'.

THE SEVENTH LETTER TO DOCTOR GIOVANNI NARDI, OF FLORENCE, A GENTLEMAN OF OUTSTANDING WORTH, MANNERS, AND LEARNING

Excellent Sir!

A long time ago I received your very pleasing letter, from which I was glad to learn that you were indeed still alive, and distinguishing yourself greatly, and working hard in our chosen field. I do not, however, know if my letter in reply to yours, together with a few books for which you asked and which I sent to you at the same time, succeeded in getting into your hands. I should be glad to become better informed at your earliest opportunity, and at the same time to know how far, pray, you have advanced with your *Noctes geniales* and the other works on which you have resolved. For I am wont to enliven my now rather inactive old age, and my spirit which scorns the trifles of everyday, by reading the best books of that kind. I again thank you most warmly for your friendly offices shown to my nephew when he was formerly in Florence. And when my other — favourite — nephew, who will bring this letter to you, has arrived in Italy, I most earnestly entreat you of your kindness to give him any help or advice which he may need from you, for in this way you will do me the greatest service. Farewell, distinguished Sir, and deign to preserve intact the memory of our friendship, as I — a supreme admirer of your virtues — promise to do in my turn.

WILLIAM HARVEY

London, 25 October, in the year 1655 of the Christian era.

THE EIGHTH LETTER TO THE DISTINGUISHED AND ELEGANT GENTLEMAN AND EXPERIENCED PHYSICIAN, JAN VLACKVELD, OF HAARLEM

Learned Sir,

There has come to me your very pleasant letter, in which you show both extreme goodwill towards myself and also exceptional industry in the cultivation of our art.

It is indeed so. Nature is nowhere wont to reveal her innermost secrets more openly than where she shows faint traces of herself away from the beaten track. Nor is there any surer route to the proper practice of medicine than if someone gives his mind over to discerning the customary law of Nature through the careful investigation of diseases that are of rare occurrence. Indeed, in practically all things it is apparently arranged that we scarcely perceive what is useful or most serviceable in them unless some are lacking in these features or have a faulty disposition. The case of the stonemason you mention is certainly an unique instance, in the elucidation of which it is possible for much discussion to arise. But it is useless for you to spur me on and for me to gird myself for some new research when I am not only ripe in years but also – let me admit – a little weary. It seems to me, indeed, that I am entitled to ask for an honourable discharge. On the other hand, it will always be a pleasure to me to see distinguished gentlemen such as yourself engaged in such worthy contest. Farewell, elegant Sir, and whatever you do continue to hold in affection

Yours respectfully,

WILLIAM HARVEY

London, 24 April, 1657.

THE only reference I have found to Vlackveld, to whom Harvey addressed the last of the eight letters, was merely a note to the effect that his doctorate thesis had been entitled *De cacochymia*.

THE ANATOMY OF THOMAS PARR

Who lived to the age of one hundred and fifty-two years and nine months, together with the observations of the renowned William Harvey and other Royal Physicians who were present.

The anatomical description here before you, curious Reader, has long been in my possession. Written down by the famous William Harvey apparently at the time to serve as a record, it was given me by his nephew the distinguished Doctor Michael Harvey, who was bound to me by ties of marriage as well as friendship. Just as I have treasured this small gift as one in which I had particular pleasure, so now because of the reputation of its author and the unusual nature of its contents, and because in some measure also of its relation to my own researches, I have come to the conclusion that it should in nowise remain unknown to the general public but should be added as an appendix to this treatise of mine.

[JOHN BETT.]

On the sixteenth day of November in the year of Our Lord one thousand six hundred and thirty-five, that day being also the anniversary of the birth of her most Serene Majesty Henrietta Maria, Queen of Great Britain, France, and Ireland.

Thomas Parr, an Englishman and a native of Winnington, a village in Shropshire, was a poor farmer of extremely advanced age. My Lord Arundel, who happened to be in those parts and whose interest had been aroused by reports of this man's incredible age, had broken his journey to see him, and then carried him off from his rural surroundings to London. Both on the journey and in his own home, my Lord looked after him with every attention, and exhibited him to the King as a remarkable phenomenon. But when he had completed 152 years and nine months of life, and had outlived nine sovereigns and enjoyed ten years of the present joyful reign, he finally failed, and died on the fourteenth day of November in the year of our Saviour 1635.

The dissection of his dead body, carried out in accordance with the commands of his most Serene Majesty, was attended by some of the foremost physicians of the time. I made the following notes.

The appearance of the body was well nourished, the chest was hairy, and the hair on the forearm was still black although the shins were hairless and smooth.

The genital organs were in good condition, the penis was neither retracted nor thin, nor was the scrotum, as is usual in old persons, distended by any watery hernia, while the testicles were large and sound – so good in fact as not to give the lie to the story commonly told of him that, after reaching his hundredth year, he was actually convicted of fornication and punished. Moreover his wife, a widow, whom he had married in his hundred and twentieth year, in reply to questions, could not deny that he had had intercourse with her exactly as other husbands do, and had kept up the practice to within twelve years of his death.

The chest was broad and full; his lungs were not spongy but, particularly on the right side, were attached to the ribs by fibrous bands. The lungs also were considerably distended with blood as is usual in pulmonary consumption (peripneumonia), so much so that before the blood was drawn off, a quantity seemed to become black. To this cause, too, I attributed the bluish colour of the face, and, a little before death, a difficulty in breathing and orthopnoea. As a result, the armpits and chest remained warm long after death. To sum up, there were clearly visible in his dead body this and other signs customarily found in those dying from suffocation. I concluded that he was suffocated, and that death was due to inability to breathe, and a similar report was given to his most Serene Majesty by all the physicians present. Later, when the blood had been drained off and wiped away from the lungs, they were seen to have a quite white and almost milky parenchyma.

The heart was large, thick, and fibrous with a considerable mass of fat around its wall and partition. The blood in the heart was blackish, liquid, and scarcely grumous. Only in the right ventricle were some clots seen.

When the sternum was dissected, the cartilages were not more osseous than in other men, but rather were flexible and soft.

The intestines were in excellent condition, fleshy and vigorous: the stomach was the same. The small intestine appeared muscular, but had some ring-shaped constrictions due to the fact that frequently he ate any kind of food both by day and night without any rules of diet or regular hours for meals. He was quite happy with half-rancid cheese and all kinds of milk dishes, brown bread, small beer, but most usually sour milk. By living frugally and roughly, and without cares, in humble circumstances, he in this way prolonged his life. He had taken a meal about the midnight shortly before his death.

The kidneys were hidden in fat and were quite large. Only on the front surface were there visible watery abscesses or small serous gatherings, one of which however was the size of a hen's egg, and contained light yellowish water in a separate cyst, and its round cavity penetrated into the kidney. To this cause some attributed the suppression of urine from which he suffered a little before his death; others, with greater probability, seem to have conjectured that the suppression of urine was due to all the serosity being drawn up into the lungs.

There was no stone in the bladder nor in the kidneys, nor was there any sign of one elsewhere.

The mesentery was very fat, and the colon and bands of fatter omentum were connected to the liver round about the fundus of the gall-bladder; the colon was attached on one side to the peritoneum, on the other to the hinder parts.

The intestines were good, although whiter on the outside as though they had been lightly boiled; inside (as was also the blood) they were stained the colour of black gore.

The spleen was remarkably small, and scarcely equal in size to a kidney. To sum up, all the internal organs seemed so sound that had he changed nothing of the routine of his former way of living, in all probability he would have delayed his death a little longer.

It was consistent to attribute the cause of death to the sudden adoption of a mode of living unnatural to him. Especially did he suffer harm from the change of air, for all his life he had enjoyed absolutely clean, rarefied, coolish, and circulating air, and therefore his diaphragm and lungs could be inflated and deflated and refreshed more freely. But life in London in particular lacks this advantage – the more so because it is full of the filth of men, animals, sewers, and other forms of squalor, in addition to which there is the not inconsiderable grime from the smoke of sulphurous coal constantly used as fuel for fires. The air in London therefore is always heavy, and in autumn particularly so, especially to a man coming from the sunny and healthy districts of Shropshire, and it could not but be particularly harmful to one who was now an enfeebled old man.

Moreover he had always hitherto existed on one kind of diet and that the simplest; therefore after he had gradually taken to a generous rich and varied diet, and stronger drink, he ruined the functions of almost all his natural parts. Finally, as the result of an increasingly sluggish stomach, less frequent expulsion of excreta, a slowing-up of the process of digestion, congestion of the liver, a less vigorous circulation of blood and numbness of his spirits, suppression of the activity of his heart which is the fount of life, constriction of the lungs which allowed no free passage of air, and the growing bulk of his body that prevented easy breathing and perspiration, it is not surprising that his soul was far from happy in such a prison and left it.

His brain was sound, and quite firm and solid to the touch. Therefore until just before his death, although he had been blind for twenty years, he could hear very well and understand what he heard, answer questions readily, and react normally to situations. He was even able to walk when lightly supported between two men. His power of memory however had failed considerably so that he had no clear remembrance of his own actions as a young man, of the public events, famous kings and leaders, wars and civil disturbances in his early youth, of customs, men, prices of goods offered for sale, or the other occurrences usually remembered by men. He remembered only his actions of most recent years. However, even in his one-hundred and thirtieth year in order to be able to earn a livelihood it was his custom to be vigorously engaged in some work on the land, and he even threshed wheat.

WILLIAM HARVEY'S LAST WILL AND TESTAMENT

A TRANSCRIPT OF THE OFFICIAL PROBATE COPY NOW IN THE WELLCOME HISTORICAL MEDICAL LIBRARY

In the name of the Almighty and Eternall God Amen. I William Harvey of London Doctor of Physick doe by these presents, make and ordaine this my last Will and Testament, in manner and forme following, Revoking hereby all former and other Will and Testament whatsoever, Imprimis I doe most humbly render my soule to him that gave it, and to my Blessed Lord, and saviour Christ Jesus, And my body to the Earth to be buried at the discreation of my Executor herein after named. The Parsonall Estate which at the time of my Decease I shall be any way possessed of either in Lawe or Equity be it in goods, household-stuffe ready moneyes, Debts, Dutyes, Arrearages of rents or any other wayes whatsoever, And whereof I shall not by this present will or by some Codicill to be hereunto annexed make a particular Guift and disposition I doe after my Debts FFuneralls, and Legacyes paid, and discharged give, and bequeath the same unto my Loving Brother Mr Eliab Harvey Merchant of London whom I make Executor of this my last Will and Testament, And whereas I have lately purch[ase]d¹ certaine Lands in Northamptonshire or thereabouts Commonly knowne by the name of Oxon Grounds and formerly belonging unto the Earle of Manchester, and certaine other grounds in Leicestershire, commonly called or knowne by the name of Barron Parke, and sometimes heretofore belonging unto Sir Henry Hastings Knight, both which purchases

---

¹ Missing letters supplied.

were made in the names of severall persons nominated, and Trusted by mee, and by two severall Deeds of Declaracion, under the hands, and seales of allpersons any wayes partyes, or privies to the said Trusts are declared to bee, ffirst upon trust, and to the intent that I should be permitted to enjoy all the rents and proffitts, and the benefit of the Collatarall security during my life, And from and after my Decease then upon trust, and for the benefitt of such person and persons, and of and for such Estate, and Estates, and interests, and for Raysing and payment[2] of such summe, and summes of money rents, Charges, Annuetyes and Yeerely payments to and for such purposes as I from time to time by any Writing or Writings to be by mee signed, and sealed in the presence of two or more Credible Witnesses, or by my last Will, and Testament, in writing, should declare Limit, direct, or Appoint, And further in Trust that the said Mannors and Lands and every part thereof together with the Collaterall security should be Assigned, Conveyed and Assured unto such persons, And for such Estates as the same should by mee be Limitted, and Directed, charged, and chargeable, Neverthelesse with all Annuetyes Rents, and summes of money by mee Limited, and Appointed if any such shall be, and in Default of such Appointment then to Eliab Harvey his heires Executors, and assignes, or to such, as hee or they shall Nominate as by the said two Deeds of Declaracion both of them bearing date, the tenth day of July in the Yeare of our Lord God 165 & 1:[3] more at Large it doth Appeare, I doe now hereby declare, Limit Direct, and Appoint that withall Convenient speed, after my decease there shalbe raised satisfyed and paid these severall summes of money Rents, Charges, and Annuityes hereinafter expressed, And likewise all such other summes of money Rents, Charges, or Annuityes, which at any time hereafter in any Codicill to be hereunto annexed shall happen to be Limited or Expressed And first I Appointed, soe much moneyes to be raised, and Laid out, upon that building which I have allready begunn to Erect within the Colledge of Physitians, in London, as will serve to ffinish the same according to the Designe allready made; Item I give and bequeath to my Loving Sister in Lawe Mrs Eliab Harvey one hundred pounds to buy something to keepe in remembrance of mee: Item I give to my Neise Mary Pratt all that Linnen, householdstuffe, and furniture

[2] 'paying' corrected to 'payment'.
[3] Sic!

which I have at Coome neer Croyden for the use of William ffoulkes, and to whom his keeping shall be Assigned after her Death, or before by me at any time, Item I give unto my Neise Mary West, and her Daughter Amy West halfe the Linnen I shall leave at London in my Chests, and Chambers, together withall my plate Excepting my Coffe pott, Item I give to my Loving sister Eliab all the other halfe of my Linnen which I shal[l][4] leave behinde mee, Item I give to my Loving sister Daniel, at Lambeth, And to every one of her children severally the summe of ffifty pounds, Item I give to my loving Cozen Mr Heneadge Finche for his paines, Counsell and advise about the Contriving of this my will, one hundred pounds, Item I give to all my little God Children, Neises and Nephewes severally to every one[5] ffifty pounds, Item I give and bequeath to the Town[e][6] of ffoulkstone where I was borne two hundred pounds to be bestowed by the advise of the Major thereof, and my Executor, for the best Use of the poore Item I give to the poore of Christ Hospitall in smithfeild thirty pounds Item I give to William Harvey my Godsonne, the sonne of my Brother Michael Harvey deceased one hundred pounds, And to his brother Michael ffifty pounds, Item I give to my Nephew Thomas Cullen and his Children one hundred pounds, And to his Brother my Godsonne William Cullen, one hundred pounds, Item I give to my Nephew John Harvey the sonne of my Loving Brother Thomas Harvey deceased two hundred pounds, Item I give to my servant John Raby for his Dilligence in my service and sicknesse twenty pounds, And to Alice Garth my servant tenne pounds, over and above what I am allready owing unto her by my Bill, which was her Mistrisses Legacy, Item I give among the poore Children of Amy Rigdon Daughter of my Loving Uncle Mr Thomas Halke, twenty pounds, Item among other my poorest Kindred one hundred pounds to be distributed at the Appointment of my Executor, Item I give among the servants of my sister Daniel at my ffuneralls ffive Pounds, And likewise among the servants of my Nephew Daniel Harvey at Coome as much, Item I give to my Cozen Mary Tomes ffiftie[7] pounds, Item I give to my Loving ffreind Mr Prestwood One hundred pounds, Item I give to every one of my Loving Brother

[4]Letter supplied.
[5]'fivety pds' (?) inserted above line.
[6]Letter supplied.
[7]'fifty pounds' inserted above the line.

Eliab his sonns, and Daughters severally ffifty pounds a peece; all which Legacyes and Guifts aforesaid are Cheifely to buy something to keepe in remembrance of mee, Item I give among the servants of my Brother, Eliab, which shalbe dwelling with him at the time of my decease tenne pounds, Furthermore I give, and bequeath unto my sister Eliabs sister, Mrs Coventry a Widowe, during her Naturall life, the Yeerely rent or summe of Twenty pounds: Item I give to my Neese Mary West during her Naturall life the yeerely rent or summe of ffourty pounds, Item I give for the Use and behoofe, and better ordering of William ffoulkes, for and during the terme of his Life unto my Neece Mary Prat, the Yeerely Rent of Tenne pounds which summe if it[8] happen my said Neece shall dye before him, I desire may bee paid to them to whom his keeping shalbee Appointed, Item I will that the twenty pounds, which I yeerely allowe him my Brother Galen Browne, may be Continued as a Legacy from his sister during his naturall life, Item I will that the Payments to Mr Samuel ffentons Children out of the proffitts of Buckhol[t][9] Lease be orderly performed as my Deare Deceased Loving Wife gave order soe long as that Lease shall stand good, Item I give unto Alice Garth during her Naturall life the Yeerely rent or summe of Twenty pounds, Item to John Raby during his Naturall life sixteene pounds Yeerely rent. All which Yeerely rents or summs to be paid halfe yeerely at the two most Usuall ffeasts in the yeere, Viz Michaelmas, and our Lady Day, Without any Deduction, for or by reason of any Mannor of Taxes, to be any way hereafter Imposed, The first payment of all the said Rents or Annuetyes respectively to beginn at such of those ffeasts which shall first happen next after my Decease; Thus I give the Remainder of my Lands unto my Loving Brother Eliab, and his heires all all[10] my Legacyes and Guifts, etc. being performed, and discharged, Touching my bookes, and householdstuffe, Pictures and Apparrell, of which I have not Already disposed I give to the Colledge of Physitians, All my Bookes, and Papers, and my best Persia long Carpet, and my blew satten Imbroydered Cushin, one paire of Brasse Andirons, with fireshovel, and Tongues of Brasse, for the Ornament of the meeting Roome I have erected for that purpose, Item I give my Velvet Gowne to my Loving ffreind Mr Doctor scarborough desiring him and my

---

[8]'shall', deleted.
[9]Letter supplied.
[10]Sic!

Loving ffreind M' Doctor Ente to looke over those scattered remnant of my poore Library, and what bookes papers, or rare Collections they shall thinke fitt, to present to the Colledge, and the rest to be sold and with the money buy better, and for their paines I give to M' Doctor Ente all the presses and shelves he please to make use of and five pounds to buy him a Ring to keepe or were in remembrance of mee And to Doctor Scarborough All my little silver Instruments of Surgery Item I give all my Chamber ffurniture Tables Bedd, Bedding, Hangings, which I have at Lambeth to my sister Daniel and her Daughter Sarah And all that at London to my Loving Sister Eliab and her Daughter or my Godsonne Eliab as Shee shall Appoint Lastly I desire my Executor to assigne over the Custody of William ffoulkes after the Death of my Neece Mary Pratt if shee happen to dye, before him, Unto the sister of the said William my Neece Mary West, Thus I have finished my last Will in three pages two of them Written with owne hand, and my name subscribed to every one, with my hand and seale to the last, William Harvey: Signed, sealed, and published as the last Will and Testament of mee William Harvey in the presence of us Edward Dering Heneage Finch Richard fflud: Francis ffinch Item I have since written a Codicill with my owne hand in a sheet of Paper to be added hereto with my name thereto subscribed and my seal[e]:[11] Item I will that the summe and Charges here specified be added, and annexed, unto my last Will, and Testament, published heretofore in the presence of Sir Edward Dering, and M' Heneage ffinch, and others, and as a Codicill by my Executor in like manner to be performed, whereby I will and bequeath to John Denne the sonne of Vincent Denne the summe of thirty Pounds, Item to my good ffreind M' Thomas Hobbs to buy something to keepe in remembrance of mee Tenne pounds, And to M' Kennersley in like manner twenty pounds, Item what moneyes shalbee due to me from M' Henry Thompson his ffees being discharged, I give to my ffreind M' Prestwood Item what money is of mine (Viz) one hundred pounds in the hands of my Cozen Rigdon, I give halfe thereof to him towards the Mariage of his neese, and the other halfe to be given to M'' Coventry for her sonne Walter when hee shall come of Yeeres And for use, my Cozen Rigdon Giving security I would hee should pay none; Item what money shalbee due to me, And Alice Garth my Servant on a

---

[11] Letter supplied.

pawne, now in the hands of of Mr Prestwood, I will, after my decease shall all be Given, my said servant for her Dilligence about me in my sicknesse and service, both Interest, and principall Item if in case it soe fall out that my good ffreind Mrs Coventry during her widowhood shall not Dyet on ffree Cost with my Brother or sister Eliab Harvey than I will and bequeath to her one hundred marke[s]^12 Yeerely during her widowhood, Item I will and bequeath to my loving Cozen Mr Heneage ffinch, (more than heretofore) to be for my Godsonne William ffinch, One hundred pounds, Item I will and bequeathe Yeerely during her Life a Rent of thirty pounds Unto Mrs Jane Nevinson Widow in case shee shall not preferre her selfe in Marriage to be paid Quarterly by even portions the first to begin at Christmas, Michaelmas our Lady Day or Midsommer which first happens after my Decease Item I give to my God-Daughter Mrs Elizabeth Glover, Daughter of my Cozen Toomes the Yeerely rent of Tenne pounds from my Decease unto the End of ffive Yeeres, Item to her Brother Mr Richard Toomes thirty pounds as a Legacy Item I give to John Cullen, sonne of Thomas Cullen, deceased all what I have formerly given his ffather, and more one hundred pounds, Item I will that what I have bequeathed to my Neece Mary West be given to her Husband my Cozen Robert West, for his Daughter Amy West, Item what should have bin to my sister Daniel deceased I will, be given my Loving Neece her Daughter in Lawe: Item I give my Cozen Mrs Mary Ranton fforty pounds to buy something to keepe in remembrance of mee, Item to my Nephewes Michael and William the sonns of my Brother Michael One hundred pounds to either of them Item all the furniture of my Chamber, and all the hangings, I give to my Godsone Mr Eliab Harvey at his Marriage, and all my red damaske ffurniture and plate to my Cozen Mary Harvey Item I give my best velvet Gowne to Doctor scarborough: William Harvey Memorandum, that upon sunday the twenty Eighth day of December in the Yeere of our Lord one Thousand six hundred ffifty six, I did againe peruse my last Will, which formerly contained three pages, and hath now this fourth page added to it, And I doe now this present sunday December 28th 1656: publish and Declare these foure pages whereof the 3 last are written with my owne hand to bee my last Will, In the presence of Heneage Finch: John Rabey:

^12Letter supplied.

INDEX

SUGGESTIONS FOR FURTHER READING

BROCK, A. J. (trans. and ed.), *Galen on the natural faculties* (London, Cambridge, 1963). Together with *Galen on the usefulness of the parts of the body*, this provides the basis for Galen's teleogical account of the functions of the body.

BYLEBYL, JEROME J., 'The School of Padua; humanistic medicine in the sixteenth century', in WEBSTER, CHARLES (ed.) *Health, medicine and mortality in the sixteenth century* (Cambridge, 1979), pp. 334–70. Discusses how anatomy rose in status in Padua.

BYLEBYL, JEROME J., 'The growth of Harvey's *De Motu Cordis*', *Bulletin of the history of medicine*, 47 (1973), pp. 427–70; Gweneth Whitteridge disagreed: '*De Motu Cordis*: written in two stages?', *Bulletin of the history of medicine*, 51 (1977), pp. 130–9; and Bylebyl's response continued on pp. 140–50.

CUNNINGHAM, ANDREW, 'Fabricius and the "Aristotle project" in anatomical teaching and research at Padua' in WEAR, A., FRENCH, R. K. & LONIE, I. M. (eds.), *The medical renaissance of the sixteenth century* (Cambridge, 1985), pp. 195–222. Analyses how Fabricius, Harvey's teacher, developed his own particular anatomical aims.

FRANK, ROBERT G., Jr, *Harvey and the Oxford Physiologists* (Berkeley, 1980). Sound and detailed analysis of English biological science after Harvey.

KEYNES, GEOFFREY, *The Life of William Harvey* (Oxford, 1978). The standard life of Harvey, brilliant and comprehensive.

O'MALLEY, C. D., *Andreas Vesalius of Brussels 1514–1564* (Berkeley, 1965). The standard work on Vesalius' anatomical work.

MAY, MARGARET (trans. and ed.), *Galen on the usefulness of the parts of the body* (2 vols, Ithaca, 1968). The Introduction gives a good account of Galen's ideas on the blood and the heart.

PAGEL, WALTER, *William Harvey's biological ideas* (Basle, 1967), and *New light on William Harvey* (Basle, 1976). Difficult but worthwhile;

places Harvey in the intellectual context of his time, including the non-'rational' and non-'scientific' aspects.

WEAR, ANDREW, 'William Harvey and the "Way of the Anatomists"', *History of Science, xxi* 1983, pp. 223–249. Shows how Harvey believed in the feasibility of an observational-anatomical basis for establishing certain knowledge.

WHITTERIDGE, GWENETH, *William Harvey and the circulation of the blood* (London and New York, 1971). Clear account seeing Harvey very much as one of the first scientists.

WHITTERIDGE, GWENETH, *The anatomical lectures of William Harvey* (Edinburgh and London, 1964). The best rendering of Harvey's difficult manuscript notes of his early anatomical lectures.

ACKNOWLEDGEMENTS

The translations by Kenneth J. Franklin of *De Motu Cordis* and *De Circulatione Sanguinis* are reprinted here by arrangement with Blackwell Scientific Publications Ltd, Oxford; the translation of *The Anatomy of Thomas Parr* by Arnold Muirhead is reprinted by kind permission of Mr Muirhead; and the transcription of *The Last Will and Testament of William Harvey* has been made by arrangement with the Wellcome Historical Medical Library.

Dr Wear would like to thank Dr Vivian Nutton for his rendering of the passage in chapter eight of *De Motu Cordis*, and for his comments on the Introduction.

ESSAYS, CRITICISM AND HISTORY
IN EVERYMAN

Essays and Poems
R. L. STEVENSON
Stevenson's hidden treasures
£4.99

The Rights of Man
THOMAS PAINE
*One of the great masterpieces
of English radicalism*
£4.99

Speeches and Letters
ABRAHAM LINCOLN
*A key document of the American
Civil War*
£5.99

Essays
FRANCIS BACON
*An excellent introduction to
Bacon's incisive wit and moral
outlook*
£4.99

Biographia Literaria
SAMUEL TAYLOR COLERIDGE
*A masterpiece of criticism,
marrying the study of literature
with philosophy*
£4.99

Selected Writings
JOHN RUSKIN
'An excellent selection'
The Guardian
£7.99

**Chesterton on Dickens:
Criticisms and Appreciations**
G. K. CHESTERTON
*A landmark in Dickens criticism,
rarely surpassed*
£4.99

History of His Own Time
BISHOP GILBERT BURNET
*A highly readable contemporary
account of the Glorious Revolution
of 1688*
£7.99

**Memoirs of the Life of Colonel
Hutchinson**
LUCY HUTCHINSON
*Biography by his wife of a man who
signed Charles I's death warrant*
£6.99

**Puritanism and Liberty: Being
the Army Debates (1647-49)
from the Clarke Manuscripts**
edited by A. S. P. Woodhouse
*A fascinating revelation of Puritan
minds in action*
£7.99

**The Embassy to Constantinople
and Other Writings**
LIUDPRAND OF CREMONA
*An insider's view of political
machinations in medieval Europe*
£5.99

All books are available from your local bookshop or direct from:
Littlehampton Book Services Cash Sales, 14 Eldon Way, Lineside Estate,
Littlehampton, West Sussex BN17 7HE *(prices are subject to change)*

To order any of the books, please enclose a cheque (in sterling) made payable to
Littlehampton Book Services, or phone your order through with credit card details (Access,
Visa or Mastercard) on 01903 721596 (24 hour answering service) stating card number
and expiry date. *(Please add £1.25 for package and postage to the total of your order.)*

In the USA, for further information and a complete catalogue call 1-800-526-2778

PHILOSOPHY AND RELIGIOUS WRITING
IN EVERYMAN

Modern Philosophy of Mind
edited by William Lyons
This unique anthology of classic readings in philosophy of mind over the last hundred years includes the writings of William James and Ludwig Wittgenstein
£6.99

Selected Writings
WILLIAM JAMES
Taking writings from James's most famous works, this edition is a comprehensive and unique selection
£6.99

The Prince and Other Political Writings
NICCOLÒ MACHIAVELLI
A clinical analysis of the dynamics of power, set in the context of Machiavelli's early political writings
£4.99

Ethics
SPINOZA
Spinoza's famous discourse on the power of understanding
£5.99

The World as Will and Idea
ARTHUR SCHOPENHAUER
New translation of abridged text, Schopenhauer's major work and key text of modern philosophy
£7.99

Utilitarianism, On Liberty, Considerations on Representative Government
J. S. MILL
Three radical works which transformed political science
£5.99

A Discourse on Method, Meditations, and Principles
RENÉ DESCARTES
Takes the theory of mind over matter into a new dimension
£5.99

An Essay Concerning Human Understanding
JOHN LOCKE
A central work in the development of modern philosophy
£5.99

Philosophical Writings
FRANCIS HUTCHESON
Comprehensive selection of Hutcheson's most influential writings
£6.99

Women Philosophers
edited by Mary Warnock
The great subjects of philosophy handled by women spanning four centuries, including Simone de Beauvoir and Iris Murdoch
£6.99

All books are available from your local bookshop or direct from:
Littlehampton Book Services Cash Sales, 14 Eldon Way, Lineside Estate,
Littlehampton, West Sussex BN17 7HE (*prices are subject to change*)

To order any of the books, please enclose a cheque (in sterling) made payable to
Littlehampton Book Services, or phone your order through with credit card details (Access,
Visa or Mastercard) on 01903 721596 (24 hour answering service) stating card number
and expiry date. (*Please add £1.25 for package and postage to the total of your order.*)

In the USA, for further information and a complete catalogue call 1-800-526-2778

CLASSIC NOVELS
IN EVERYMAN

The Time Machine
H. G. WELLS

*One of the books which defined
'science fiction' – a compelling
and tragic story of a brilliant
and driven scientist*
£3.99

Oliver Twist
CHARLES DICKENS

*Arguably the best-loved of
Dickens's novels. With all the
original illustrations*
£4.99

Barchester Towers
ANTHONY TROLLOPE

*The second of Trollope's
Chronicles of Barsetshire,
and one of the funniest of all
Victorian novels*
£4.99

The Heart of Darkness
JOSEPH CONRAD

*Conrad's most intense, subtle,
compressed, profound and
proleptic work*
£3.99

Tess of the d'Urbervilles
THOMAS HARDY

*The powerful, poetic classic
of wronged innocence*
£3.99

Wuthering Heights and Poems
EMILY BRONTË

*A powerful work of genius – one of
the great masterpieces of literature*
£3.99

Pride and Prejudice
JANE AUSTEN

*Proposals, rejections, infidelities,
elopements, happy marriages –
Jane Austen's most popular novel*
£2.99

North and South
ELIZABETH GASKELL

*A novel of hardship, passion
and hard-won wisdom amidst the
conflicts of the industrial revolution*
£4.99

The Newcomes
W. M. THACKERAY

*An exposé of Victorian polite
society by one of the nineteenth-
century's finest novelists*
£6.99

Adam Bede
GEORGE ELIOT

*A passionate rural drama enacted
at the turn of the eighteenth
century*
£5.99

All books are available from your local bookshop or direct from:
Littlehampton Book Services Cash Sales, 14 Eldon Way, Lineside Estate,
Littlehampton, West Sussex BN17 7HE (*prices are subject to change*)

To order any of the books, please enclose a cheque (in sterling) made payable to
Littlehampton Book Services, or phone your order through with credit card details (Access,
Visa or Mastercard) on 01903 721596 (24 hour answering service) stating card number
and expiry date. (*Please add £1.25 for package and postage to the total of your order.*)

In the USA, for further information and a complete catalogue call 1-800-526-2778

CLASSIC FICTION
IN EVERYMAN

The Impressions of Theophrastus Such
GEORGE ELIOT
An amusing collection of character sketches, and the only paperback edition available
£5.99

Frankenstein
MARY SHELLEY
A masterpiece of Gothic terror in its original 1818 version
£3.99

East Lynne
MRS HENRY WOOD
A classic tale of melodrama, murder and mystery
£7.99

Holiday Romance and Other Writings for Children
CHARLES DICKENS
Dickens's works for children, including 'The Life of Our Lord' and 'A Child's History of England', with original illustrations
£5.99

The Ebb-Tide
R. L. STEVENSON
A compelling study of ordinary people in extreme circumstances
£4.99

The Three Impostors
ARTHUR MACHEN
The only edition available of this cult thriller
£4.99

Mister Johnson
JOYCE CARY
The only edition available of this amusing but disturbing twentieth-century tale
£5.99

The Jungle Book
RUDYARD KIPLING
The classic adventures of Mowgli and his friends
£3.99

Glenarvon
LADY CAROLINE LAMB
The only edition available of the novel which throws light on the greatest scandal of the early nineteenth century – the infatuation of Caroline Lamb with Lord Byron
£6.99

Twenty Thousand Leagues Under the Sea
JULES VERNE
Scientific fact combines with fantasy in this prophetic tale of underwater adventure
£4.99

FOREIGN LITERATURE IN TRANSLATION
IN EVERYMAN

A Hero of Our Time
MIKHAIL LERMONTOV
*The Byronic adventures of
a Russian army officer*
£5.99

L'Assommoir
ÉMILE ZOLA
*One of the most successful novels
of the nineteenth century and one
of the most scandalous*
£6.99

Poor Folk and **The Gambler**
FYODOR DOSTOYEVSKY
*These two short works of doomed
passion are among Dostoyevsky's
quintessential best. Combination
unique to Everyman*
£4.99

Yevgeny Onegin
ALEXANDER PUSHKIN
*Pushkin's novel in verse is Russia's
best-loved literary work. It contains some of the loveliest Russian
poetry ever written*
£5.99

The Three-Cornered Hat
ANTONIO PEDRO DE ALARCÓN
*A rollicking farce and one of
the world's greatest masterpieces
of humour. Available only in
Everyman*
£4.99

Notes from Underground
and **A Confession**
FYODOR DOSTOYEVSKY *and*
LEV TOLSTOY
*Russia's greatest novelists ruthlessly
tackle the subject of their mid-life
crises. Combination unique to
Everyman*
£4.99

Selected Stories
ANTON CHEKHOV
edited and revised by Donald
Rayfield
*Masterpieces of compression and
precision. Selection unique to
Everyman*
£7.99

Selected Writings
VOLTAIRE
*A comprehensive edition of
Voltaire's best writings. Selection
unique to Everyman*
£6.99

Fontamara
IGNAZIO SILONE
*'A beautifully composed tragedy.
Fontamara is as fresh now, and as
moving, as it must have been when
first published.'* London Standard.
Available only in Everyman
£4.99

All books are available from your local bookshop or direct from:
Littlehampton Book Services Cash Sales, 14 Eldon Way, Lineside Estate,
Littlehampton, West Sussex BN17 7HE *(prices are subject to change)*

To order any of the books, please enclose a cheque (in sterling) made payable to
Littlehampton Book Services, or phone your order through with credit card details (Access,
Visa or Mastercard) on 01903 721596 (24 hour answering service) stating card number
and expiry date. *(Please add £1.25 for package and postage to the total of your order.)*

In the USA, for further information and a complete catalogue call 1-800-526-2778

POETRY
IN EVERYMAN